The Brompton Hospital
Guide to
Chest Physiotherapy

D. V. Gaskell MCSP
and
B. A. Webber MCSP

The Brompton Hospital Guide to Chest Physiotherapy

Fourth Edition
Revised by B. A. Webber

Blackwell Scientific Publications
OXFORD LONDON EDINBURGH
BOSTON MELBOURNE

© The Brompton Hospital 1977, 1980

Published by
Blackwell Scientific Publications
Editorial offices:
Osney Mead, Oxford OX2 oEL
8 John Street, London WC1N 2ES
9 Forrest Road, Edinburgh EH1 2QH
52 Beacon Street, Boston
    Massachusetts 02108, USA
99 Barry Street, Carlton
    Victoria 3053, Australia

First published as *Physiotherapy for Medical
and Surgical Thoracic Conditions* 1960
Revised reprints 1962, 1964, 1967
Second edition (under present title) 1973
Revised reprint 1974
Reprinted 1975
Third edition 1977
Reprinted 1979
Fourth edition 1980
Reprinted 1982

Printed and bound in Great Britain at
the Alden Press, Oxford

DISTRIBUTORS

USA
  Blackwell Mosby Book Distributors
  11830 Westline Industrial Drive
  St Louis, Missouri 63141

Canada
  Blackwell Mosby Book Distributors
  120 Melford Drive, Scarborough
  Ontario M1B 2X4

Australia
  Blackwell Scientific Book Distributors
  214 Berkeley Street, Carlton
  Victoria 3053

British Library
Cataloguing in Publication Data

Gaskell, Diana Vaughan
  The Brompton Hospital guide to chest
  physiotherapy.
  –4th ed.
  1. Chest; Physical therapy –
  I. Title II. Webber, Barbara Anne
  617'.54   RC731

  ISBN 0–632–00576–9

Contents

Preface to second edition

This book is intended as a practical guide for physiotherapists and others concerned with the treatment of chest conditions. It is derived from the booklet *Physiotherapy for Medical and Surgical Thoracic Conditions* originally compiled at the Brompton Hospital in 1960.

The development of physiotherapeutic techniques in the treatment of chest disease was begun at the Brompton Hospital in 1934 by the late Miss Winifred Linton, FCSP(HON), who became superintendent physiotherapist at that time. These techniques have subsequently been further developed and modified as advances in the medical and surgical management of chest disease have occurred, and more understanding of the physiology of normal respiration has been gained.

The basic techniques of breathing exercises and postural drainage and an outline of the relevant anatomy are described. Physiotherapy for a wide variety of medical and surgical cardio-thoracic conditions is included. There are also sections on the treatment of patients undergoing artificial ventilation and an account of the uses of intermittent positive pressure breathing as a valuable adjunct to physiotherapy.

In order to make intelligent use of the techniques described in the following text, the physiotherapist must have a detailed knowledge of the anatomical mechanism of respiration and the physiology of gaseous exchange. A basic knowledge of the interpretation of electrocardiographs is also useful. This additional knowledge can be obtained from the appropriate text books.

It is important to appreciate that the physiotherapist is a member of a team which includes nurses, technicians and the patient, all under the direction of a physician or surgeon. The more each person is cognisant of the others' contribution, and the more their efforts are co-ordinated, the better will be the results.

The authors would like to thank Dr M.A.Branthwaite, MRCP, FFARCS, for assistance and advice given during the preparation of this book. They are also grateful to Professor R.J.Last, FRCS, and to Mrs S.A.Hyde, MCSP, for their helpful suggestions.

D.V.G.
B.A.W.

Preface to fourth edition

Owing to other commitments Miss Gaskell has left the revision of *The Brompton Hospital Guide to Chest Physiotherapy* to me. I would like to thank her for reading the new manuscript.

Many changes have been made in this new edition to keep pace with recent developments in treatment methods. Appropriate references are included at the end of each chapter and a list of textbooks is added. Readers are reminded that this is a practical guide to chest physiotherapy and is intended to be used with a background knowledge of physiology and pathology gained from comprehensive texts.

Sections on the basic interpretation of lung sounds and chest radiographs have been added. Although the chapter on radiographs may appear lengthy in this slim book, it was felt that it may be helpful to physiotherapists as available texts are either very detailed or too slight.

I am grateful to members of the medical staff at the Brompton Hospital and the physiotherapy staff, particularly Miss A.J.Davis and Miss J.A.Pryor, for their help in the preparation of this edition.

B.A.W.

1 Anatomy of the thoracic cage and lungs

Movements of the rib cage

An understanding of the normal mechanism of respiration is essential before teaching breathing exercises. This mechanism depends not only on the anatomy of the respiratory muscles, but in particular the ribs and their articulations in the thoracic cage. To quote Professor R.J.Last[1]: 'The ribs are to breathe with.'

During respiration, changes in volume of the thoracic cage are brought about in three diameters.

The antero-posterior diameter of the thorax is increased by elevation of the ribs. The manubrium of the sternum is fixed by a primary cartilaginous joint to the first costal cartilage and the manubrium and the first ribs are fixed to each other and move together as one. As the manubrium is elevated its lower border projects anteriorly. This border articulates by a hinge joint to the body of the sternum, movement occurring at this joint as the body of the sternum rises with the ribs. (If this joint becomes ankylosed, thoracic expansion is virtually lost.)

The costal cartilages of the second to seventh ribs articulate with the sternum by a synovial joint and the eighth, ninth and tenth costal cartilages articulate with the cartilage above by a synovial joint.

The ribs slope downwards from their attachment to the vertebral column towards the sternum, at an angle of 45°. Rotation of the neck of the ribs occurs at all twelve costo-vertebral joints and this results in elevation or depression of the anterior ends of the ribs.

As a result of the obliquity of the ribs, elevation of the sternum carries it forwards and thus the antero-posterior diameter of the thorax is increased. This up and down movement of the body of the sternum and the ribs attached to it, is often termed the 'pump-handle movement'.

The transverse diameter of the thorax is increased in two ways, one passive and the other active. The passive increase is due to the shape of the ribs and the axis round which they hinge during inspiration. The axis is not transverse across the body, but passes through the head and tubercle of

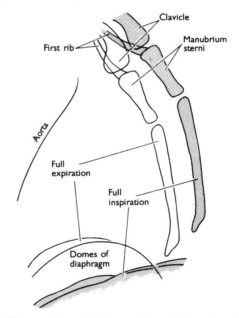

Fig. 1. *Lateral X-ray view of the thoracic cavity of a healthy young male, showing maximum excursion simultaneously of the chest wall and of the diaphragm. From R.J.Last.[1]*

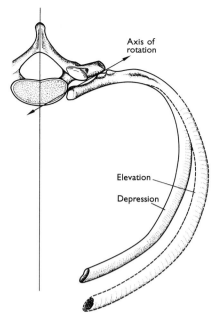

Axis of rotation

Elevation

Depression

Fig. 2. *The axis of rotation of a rib. From R.J.Last.*[1]

each rib obliquely backwards from the mid-line (figs. 1 & 2). Therefore the downward sloping rib is not only elevated antero-posteriorly but also laterally. This lateral spread of the ribs increases from the fifth rib downwards because the costal cartilages become progressively more oblique. It does not occur in the upper four pairs, as their costal cartilages are too short to allow such separation from the mid line.

The active increase in transverse diameter is brought about by the 'bucket-handle' movement of the lower ribs. These ribs rotate about an axis that passes through the anterior and posterior extremity of each, like lifting up the fallen handle from the side of a bucket.

This movement can occur because the articular surfaces of the seventh to tenth costo-vertebral joints are flat; the tubercles

of these ribs can move up and down, in addition to the rotation occurring at the neck of the rib.

The vertical diameter of the thorax is increased by descent of the diaphragm.

The muscles of inspiration

The most important muscle of inspiration is the diaphragm. It is a bi-domed muscle, its fibres originating from the sternum, the lower ribs and the upper lumbar vertebrae. In full expiration the right dome rises to the level of the 4th intercostal space (nipple level), while the left dome is at the level of the 5th rib. The central tendon is level with the lower end of the sternum. In quiet inspiration, only the domes of the diaphragm descend and there is no movement of the central tendon. In a deeper breath, further descent of the domes below the level of the central tendon can depress the central tendon from the level of the 8th thoracic vertebra to the 9th thoracic vertebra. This stretches the mediastinum and no further descent of the central tendon is possible. The diaphragm will only descend if the abdominal wall relaxes. With further contraction of the muscle (i.e. maximum inspiration) the outer fibres evert the ribs of the costal margin in the 'bucket-handle' movement.

The 12th rib, held down by quadratus lumborum is not elevated with the other ribs. This fixes the posterior fibres of the diaphragm and increases the vertical dia-meter of the thorax.

The fibres of the external intercostal muscles pass obliquely downwards and forwards between the ribs. When the muscles contract, they lift the ribs in a powerful inspiratory movement. The external inter-costal muscle fibres cease and become a membrane between the costal cartilages. These cartilages slope in the opposite obliquity to the ribs, and the part of the internal intercostal muscle that lies between these costal cartilages elevates them when its fibres shorten.

The accessory muscles of inspiration can be brought into action to produce an increase in ventilation. The sternomastoids, with the help of the scalene muscles, elevate the thoracic inlet, while the head extensor muscles fix the head in extension. If the arms are fixed in abduction, the muscles attaching the upper limbs to the trunk are inspiratory; these are the pectoral muscles, serratus anterior, and the costal fibres of latissimus dorsi.

The muscles of expiration

During quiet or forced expiration the diaphragm is completely passive, its relaxed fibres being elongated by pressure from below.

Depression of the ribs and sternum is passive during quiet expiration. It is brought about by the elastic recoil of the chest wall and lungs. To produce a forced expiration the lateral fibres of the internal intercostal muscles contract, depressing the ribs. The thoracic cage is also depressed by the downward pull of the rectus abdominis and oblique abdominal muscles, on the ribs; at the same time the abdominal muscles elevate the diaphragm by raising the intra-abdominal pressure.

Structure of airways and alveoli

It is not intended to give a detailed description of the anatomy and physiology of the respiratory system, but a few facts concerning the structure of the airways are described to assist the understanding of some mechanisms involved in respiratory physiotherapy.

The *trachea* extends from the cricoid cartilage (lower border of C6) to the bifurcation of the main bronchi at the level of the angle of Louis (upper border of T5). It is lined by ciliated columnar epithelium containing plentiful mucus-secreting glands and goblet cells. The wall is a fibro-elastic membrane whose patency is maintained by C-shaped rings of cartilage. The gaps lie posteriorly and are closed by a sheet of muscle which plays an important part in the efficacy of coughing and huffing.

The *bronchi* are airways which have cartilage in their walls. The proximal five generations have abundant cartilage, but the fifth to fifteenth generations are smaller bronchi with scattered plates of cartilage throughout the walls. The walls of the bronchi also contain fibrous tissue with a capillary network and longitudinal bands of elastic fibres. They are lined by layers of epithelium containing numerous mucus-secreting glands, goblet cells and ciliated cells.

Bronchioli are airways distal to the last plate of cartilage and proximal to the alveolar region. They are about 1 mm or less in diameter. Their walls are composed of smooth muscle fibres arranged circularly and lined by epithelium containing some mucous glands, goblet cells and ciliated cells. The distal bronchioli are lined with only one layer of epithelium and have very few mucus-secreting cells.

In massive collapse of a lobe the large bronchi are inherently rigid enough to remain patent, whereas the walls of the small bronchi and bronchioli collapse and come into apposition.

All bronchioli eventually reach a point

where alveoli open into the lumen. This part is known as the *respiratory bronchiole*. *Ciliated cells* appear in the epithelial lining of the airways from the level of the respiratory bronchiole and are responsible for shifting mucus and other particles from this level to the larynx. The cilia beat in a liquid layer known as the periciliary layer and the viscous secretions that make up sputum rest on the surface of this liquid (fig. 3). When a patient is dehydrated, the periciliary layer becomes reduced or absent and the cilia become entangled in the mucus, making the clearance mechanism ineffective. A *terminal bronchiole* is defined as the airway immediately proximal to the respiratory bronchiole (fig. 4). The terminal bronchioli contain no cilia and no mucus-secreting glands or goblet cells.

An *acinus* is the area of lung distal to the terminal bronchiole and includes several generations of respiratory bronchioli (up to

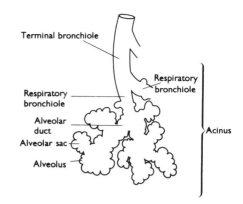

Fig. 4. *Respiratory bronchiole.*

8), alveolar ducts and alveoli. An acinus is approximately 0·5–1 cm in diameter.

A recent estimate of the total number of alveoli in the average adult lung is thought to be in the region of 300 million.

An *alveolus* is an air sac consisting of a single layer of flat cells and a network of fine elastic fibres. A rich network of capilaries surrounds it.

Alveolar pores are openings that exist in the alveolar walls of the human lung allowing drift of air from alveolus to alveolus and thereby from lobule to lobule and segment to segment, without using the airways. This phenomenon is known as *collateral air drift* and by providing alternative pathways for the passage of air, collapse of segments of a lung distal to a plugged bronchus does not necessarily occur. The pleura prevents drift of air between the lobes of the lungs.

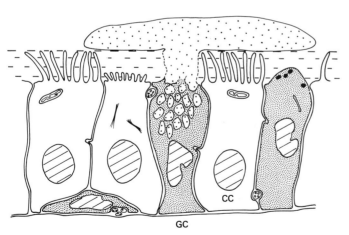

Fig. 3. *Diagrammatic representation of cells in lining epithelium, fluid layer in which cilia beat, and thick mucus that may be on tips of cilia. GC: goblet cell; CC: ciliated cell. By courtesy of Professor Lynne Reid.*[2]

References

1. LAST R.J. (1972) *Anatomy, Regional and Applied*. 5th edition. Churchill, London.
2. REID L. (1973) Development and anatomy of the lung. *Medicine* **13**, 811.

2 Chest radiographs— basic interpretation

Interpretation of the radiograph is an important part of the assessment of chest disease, and although the physiotherapist will depend on the medical staff to interpret the finer details, a basic understanding is valuable.

The radiograph is a photographic negative where the degree of blackening depends on the amount of absorption of X-rays by the structures in their passage. The more solid structures such as bone, fluid and soft tissues absorb more of the X-rays and appear relatively white, while the less solid structures containing air appear relatively black.

The radiograph should always be examined systematically to avoid missing useful information.

Postero-anterior or antero-posterior view

In the postero-anterior (PA) or antero-posterior (AP) film the following details are observed:

1 The *name*, *sex* of the patient and *date* of the film.

2 *Positioning*. The patient should be positioned centrally in relation to the film. If accurately centred, the distance between the medial end of each clavicle and the lateral edge of the vertebral body over which it lies should be equal. Inequality of this distance denotes rotation of the patient and can lead to misinterpretation of the film.

3 *Exposure*. It is important that the film is neither over nor under exposed. The outline of the vertebral bodies should be just visible through the central mediastinal shadow. It is often useful to compare a recent radiograph with previous films, but differences in exposure must be taken into account.

4 *Soft tissue shadows*. Breast shadows may obscure the lower lung zones except at the costophrenic angles. The unilateral absence of breast shadow resulting from mastectomy can be noted. Subcutaneous (surgical) emphysema may be seen as darker areas in between layers of connective tissue in the chest wall. Post-operatively it may track along the fascial planes outlining the pectoral muscles and neurovascular bundles in the axilla. If the air leaks into the mediastinum, it may seep up into the neck.

It is important that external articles such as dressings, electrodes or an oxygen mask and tubing should not be misinterpreted as intrathoracic shadows.

5 *Bony structures*. The rib cage and spinal column are observed for deformity, the presence of cervical rib, rib fractures and previous rib resection for thoracotomy. Notching of ribs is characteristic of coarctation of the aorta.

Osteoporosis of the bony structures should also be noted. The ribs normally slope symmetrically downwards and forwards from the vertebral column. In scoliosis they slope more steeply on the side of the concavity. Apart from spinal deformity, steeply sloping ribs with narrowed intercostal spaces indicate diminished lung volume on that side, from old or recent disease.

The ribs are more horizontal than normal and the intercostal spaces widened when the chest is hyperinflated as in emphysema, asthma or with large pleural effusions.

6 *Trachea*. The shadow of the trachea

normally lies centrally with the lower third deviating slightly to the right. Provided the patient has been positioned centrally, any greater deviation of the trachea is helpful in assessing mediastinal shift.

7 *Heart shadow.* The heart shadow is observed for abnormality of outline and 'true' enlargement.

The transverse diameter of the heart is normally less than 50% of the total transverse diameter of the rib cage. In the standard postero-anterior film the patient stands facing and close to the film and the shadow of the heart is approximately the true size. In an antero-posterior film, taken when the patient is confined to bed, the film is placed behind the patient and heart size becomes exaggerated due to geometrical magnification.

In the majority of normal persons, one-third of the heart lies to the right of the mid-line and two-thirds to the left, but one-quarter to three-quarters is accepted as normal. In emphysema, the heart tends to be narrow and vertical partly as a result of the low position of the diaphragm.

8 *The diaphragm and costo-phrenic angles.* The two hemidiaphragms should be rounded, smooth, sharply defined shadows, with the level of the right dome being normally 2 cm higher than the left in all phases of respiration. If, however, there is a large amount of gas in the stomach or colon, the left dome may be elevated. On a radiograph taken in full inspiration, the right hemidiaphragm is intersected by the shadow of the anterior part of the sixth rib (fig. 5a).

In emphysema the domes of the diaphragm are typically low and flattened. The diaphragm is considered low if it is below the anterior end of the right sixth intercostal space. Elevation of one dome of the

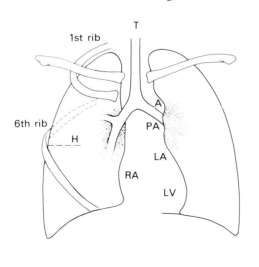

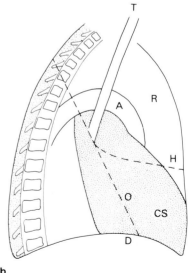

a

b

Fig. 5. *Diagram of anatomical features on a normal chest radiograph: (a) PA and (b) lateral views. T: trachea; A: aorta; PA: pulmonary artery; LA: left atrial appendage; LV: left ventricle; RA: right atrium; D: diaphragm; H: horizontal fissure; O: oblique fissure; R: retrosternal air space; CS: cardiac shadow.*

diaphragm may result from damage to the phrenic nerve or to the muscle itself, or from compression of lung, for example by pleural fibrosis. In the normal radiograph the costophrenic angles should be acute, sharply defined and symmetrical.

9 *Hilar shadows.* The areas of increased density in the medial part of the central portion of the lung fields are known as the hilar shadows. They consist of the pulmonary arteries, their branches and the pulmonary veins. The pulmonary vessels visible throughout the lung fields fan out from the hila. In a normal radiograph the left hilum is partly obscured by the main pulmonary artery and it lies at a slightly higher level than the right hilum.

Enlargement of both hila is seen when diffuse pulmonary disease leads to an increase in pulmonary artery pressure and also when there is bilateral hilar lymph node enlargement as in sarcoidosis. Enlargement of one hilum is suspicious of malignant disease. Elevation of one or both hila can result from apical fibrosis and unilateral depression of the hilum is associated with collapse of the lower lobe.

10 *Lung fields.* The upper, middle and lower zones of the lung fields are compared, one side with the other, for any difference in shadowing. In a normal radiograph the lung markings which are produced by the pulmonary vessels extend over the entire lung fields to the rib cage. Valuable information can be obtained from study of the vessels in the lungs. In the upright position the size of the blood vessels is normally greater in the lower half of the lung than the upper half.

Absence or diminution of the peripheral markings are important signs in emphysema. The habit of scanning the lung vessels from the periphery towards the hilum, helps to concentrate attention on any avascular areas such as pneumothorax at the periphery, or bullae within the lung field.

The bronchi are not usually visible beyond 2–3 cm from the hilum on a normal radiograph unless they are viewed end-on. A bronchus is then seen as a ring-like area of increase density with a central translucency, whereas a blood vessel seen end-on appears as a round solid shadow. This is distinguished from an intrapulmonary nodule by identification of the vessel leading into and out of the opacity.

When the bronchial walls are grossly thickened with disease and if they are also dilated as in bronchiectasis, they may be seen as parallel line shadows.

The horizontal fissure which divides the right upper lobe from the middle lobe is seen in 50–60 % of normal persons as a fine hair-like line at the level of the sixth rib in the mid-axillary line extending horizontally to the level of the third or fourth costal cartilage anteriorly. In the normal, the outer end may curve downwards slightly. Deviation of this fissure is a guide to shrinkage of the right lung resulting from lobar collapse or fibrosis (fig. 6). The right and left oblique fissures are not normally visible on the postero-anterior film.

Lateral view

A lateral chest radiograph is helpful in accurately identifying the position of an abnormality.

1 *Oblique fissure.* In a normal film the oblique fissure appears as a thin line which extends from the body of the fourth thoracic vertebra across the hilum and down to meet the diaphragm at the anterior third (fig. 5b). With collapse of the lower lobe the oblique fissure is drawn downwards and posteriorly,

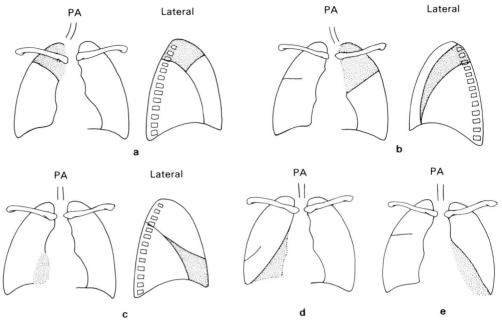

Fig. 6. *Diagrammatic representation of lobar collapse seen on radiographs. (a) Right upper lobe collapse. (b) Left upper lobe collapse. (c) Middle lobe collapse. (d) Right lower lobe collapse. (e) Left lower lobe collapse.*

but with upper lobe collapse the fissure balloons upwards.

2 *Horizontal fissure.* This fissure lies horizontally at the level of the centre of the right hilum and may curve downwards slightly at the anterior end.

3 *Hemidiaphragms.* The left hemidiaphragm is distinguished by the presence of the stomach gas bubble.

4 *Retrosternal air space.* The relatively transradiant area behind the sternum and in front of the heart shadow is often enlarged in severe emphysema as a result of hyperinflation of the lungs.

Common abnormalities

Atelectasis or collapse. Collapse of a lobe is usually evident from the shift of landmarks such as the fissures, mediastinum and blood vessels. Characteristic shadows may be cast by the collapsed lobe itself (fig. 6). Solid structures, such as the heart and diaphragm, which rest against aerated lung, normally appear to have a well-defined margin. When a lobe collapses and the air within is absorbed, the clear margin of the adjacent structure disappears. If an upper lobe is collapsed the position of the trachea and mediastinal shadow may shift slightly towards the side of the collapse. If the lower lobe is collapsed there may be slight elevation and loss of definition of the diaphragm and displacement of the heart to that side. The hilar shadow appears smaller on the side of a lobar collapse, and as the lobe adjacent to the collapsed lobe occupies more space than normal, the vessel markings are more spread out.

8

The middle lobe lies up against the right heart shadow. On the postero-anterior film the right heart border disappears with collapse of the middle lobe and on a right lateral film it appears as a triangular shadow between the horizontal and oblique fissures. Similarly, the left heart border is lost when the lingula is collapsed. Left lower lobe collapse is characterised by a triangular shadow superimposed on the heart shadow with a well-defined straight line at the lateral margin. With right lower lobe collapse a similar triangular shadow may be superimposed on the right heart, or the shrunken lobe may lie behind the heart shadow. The horizontal fissure is pulled downwards.

Complete collapse of a lung occurs if there is total occlusion of the main bronchus. The lung appears opaque and shrunken as the air within becomes absorbed and the trachea and mediastinum shift *towards* the affected side (fig. 7a).

Consolidation. A consolidated lobe is one in which the alveolar air has been replaced by fluid, cells or cellular exudate and it has an opaque appearance on a radiograph. The dimensions of the lobe remain approximately normal. Patent bronchi may be visible as an air bronchogram.

Pleural effusions. A small pleural effusion may cause blunting of the costophrenic angle. A large effusion casts an opaque shadow with a curved upper edge rising towards the axilla. A very large effusion can obliterate one side of the chest and may produce mediastinal shift *away* from the affected side (fig. 7b).

If fluid is suspected in the pleural space, but is not grossly evident on the ordinary film, it may become apparent if a film is taken with the patient lying on the suspected side (lateral decubitus film). Free fluid moves to the most dependent position. In the supine position the fluid in the most dependent part is lying posteriorly and therefore appears as a generalised haziness over the whole of one lung. In the erect position the fluid will shift to lie in the costophrenic angle and a clear view of the lung will be obtained.

Occasionally fluid is visible in the horizontal fissure on a PA or AP film, but a lateral film is often required to recognise effusions localised within the fissures.

Pleural fluid only appears with a horizontal upper border when air is also present in the pleural space.

Pneumothorax. A large pneumothorax can

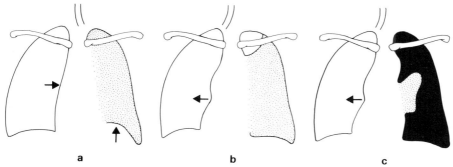

Fig. 7. *Diagrammatic representation of abnormalities seen on radiographs. (a) Total left lung collapse. (b) Large left pleural effusion (c) Large left pneumothorax. Arrows show direction of mediastinal shift and the change of position of the diaphragm.*

9

be identified easily as a clear zone with no vascular markings and a shrunken underlying lung. There will be mediastinal shift *away* from the affected side (fig. 7c). When a pneumothorax is small, a fine line shadow marks the edge of the lung and may be difficult to see. A radiograph taken at full expiration makes identification easier by increasing the relative size of the pneumothorax and decreasing the air content (blackness) of the lung.

Bullae. A bulla is a transradiant area containing no vessel markings and with a fine white line of demarcation. Very large bullae cause compression of the unaffected lung tissue with crowding of vascular markings.

Lung abscess. A lung abscess appears as a rounded shadow, and may have a fluid level. A lateral film may be necessary to determine the exact position of the abscess.

Special radiographic investigations

Tomography. This is a special radiographic technique in which a series of radiographs can be obtained at different planes through the lung. It is useful in defining tumours and cavities by blurring of the overlying structures such as ribs.

Fluoroscopy. Screening, or fluoroscopy, is a method of observing movement of the diaphragm during the respiratory cycle. If paralysis of one side of the diaphragm is suspected the 'sniff' test is carried out. When the patient sniffs the paralysed hemidiaphragm rises, whereas the normal diaphragm moves sharply downwards. This paradoxical upward movement of the paralysed diaphragm is caused by the increased intra-abdominal pressure. Flouroscopy is also used to identify cardiac abnormalities and shift of the mediastinum by air trapping as may occur if a peanut is inhaled into a bronchus.

Pulmonary angiography. A radio-opaque substance is injected into the bloodstream and radiographs are taken as it passes through the pulmonary circulation, heart and aorta. This is a valuable procedure in the diagnosis of pulmonary embolism in conjunction with radio-isotope studies.

Bronchography. A radio-opaque contrast medium is introduced into the trachea, usually under local anaesthesia, either by a nasal catheter or a catheter through the cricothyroid membrane. By varied positioning of the patient the bronchopulmonary segments are lined by the contrast medium. Lateral, oblique and postero-anterior radiographs are taken.

This investigation is used to confirm the diagnosis if bronchiectasis is suspected. The exact site and extent of the bronchial disease can be established (p. 52).

References

1. SHANKS S.C. & KERLEY P. (1973) *A Textbook of X-Ray Diagnosis.* 4th edition, Vol. III. Lewis, London.
2. SIMON G. (1971) *Principles of Chest X-Ray Diagnosis.* 3rd edition. Butterworths, London.
3. SIMON G. (1974) How to look at a chest radiograph. *British Journal of Hospital Medicine* **12,** 707.
4. GODWIN R.J. (1978) Chest X-Rays after abdominal surgery. *Physiotherapy* **64,** (2), 34.

3 Lung sounds

Auscultation is the art of listening to sounds. Listening to and interpreting lung sounds, or the absence of lung sounds, can aid the physiotherapist in the assessment of the patient both before and after treatment.

Coarse changes in lung sounds may be detected by the unaided ear, but a stethoscope will help to localise the source. The stethoscope consists of a diaphragm or bell connected by a length of tubing to two ear pieces. The ear pieces should point slightly forward as they enter the ear and should fit comfortably, but firmly.

An area of one side of the chest wall is compared with the equivalent area on the other side. The patient is asked to breathe deeply, but not noisily, through his mouth. This minimises any sounds which may be produced in his nose.

The classification of lung sounds follows the nomenclature originally stated by Laënnec in the early nineteenth century when he divided them into the universally accepted normal and bronchial breath sounds. Further divisions have been defined in various ways, but the following can be used as a guideline.

1 *Normal breath sounds* are faint and low pitched. The inspiratory sound is followed, without a pause, by the expiratory sound. The expiratory sound soon becomes inaudible and appears comparatively short.

2 *Bronchial breath sounds* are the sounds which resemble the noise of breathing heard through the stethoscope held over the trachea, but they are abnormal when heard over the chest wall. These sounds are the noise breathing makes in the bronchi and under normal circumstances are dampened and lost by the buffering effect of the air-filled alveoli. Areas of consolidation and atelectasis facilitate the transmission of breath sounds to the surface. The harsh sound can be heard throughout inspiration and expiration and there is a pause between the two phases with the expiratory phase being as long or longer than that of inspiration. If the bronchi are not patent in an area of consolidation or atelectasis, breath sounds will be absent as there is no direct route of transmission.

3 *Reduced breath sounds* are not necessarily synonomous with reduced ventilation of that part of the lung. Air entry may be normal, that is the bronchi may be patent, but the breath sounds diminished by intervening pathology of the lung or pleura.

4 Crackles and wheezes are added, or adventitious sounds.

(a) *Crackles* are discontinuous or explosive sounds often confined to inspiration and thought to be produced by alveoli, bronchioles or bronchi suddenly opening up under an explosive equalisation of gas pressure. They may also be attributed to the bubbling of bronchial secretions in the airways as in bronchitis, bronchiectasis and pulmonary oedema; coughing may cause disappearance of these sounds or alter their distribution. Crackles are also heard in the absence of excess secretions as in fibrosing alveolitis.

Pleural crackles (pleural rub) are usually localised to a small area and do not disappear or alter with coughing. They are due to friction between the parietal and visceral pleura, indicating a lesion.

(b) *Wheezes* are musical notes produced as air flows through narrowed air passages on the point of collapse and consequently first become apparent during expiration when the airways shorten and narrow. As further narrowing takes place, they are also apparent during inspiration.

5 *Stridor* is the crowing noise emanating from the larynx or trachea on inspiration caused by an obstruction in this region.

6 Further information may be gained from *percussion*. This is the firm tapping of the thoracic wall in order to produce sound vibrations from which the nature of the underlying structures can be detected.

Percussion over a normal chest gives a characteristic resonant note. In pathological conditions the noise may become more or less resonant varying from hyper-resonance to complete dullness. A pneumothorax conveys a hyper-resonant note, but over collapsed or consolidated areas the percussion note is dull and if fluid is present it is 'stony dull'.

References

1. FORGACS P. (1978) *Lung Sounds*. Ballière Tindall, London.
2. CROFTON J. & DOUGLAS A. (1975) *Respiratory Diseases*. 2nd edition. Blackwell Scientific Publications, Oxford.
3. BASKETT P.J.F. (1971) The clinical assessment of the respiratory system by the physiotherapist, including reference to the use of the stethoscope. *Physiotherapy* 57, 319.

4 Breathing exercises and postural drainage

BREATHING EXERCISES

Aims

To obtain the best possible lung function by:
1 Promoting a normal relaxed pattern of breathing, where possible.
2 Teaching controlled breathing with the minimum amount of effort.
3 Assisting with removal of secretions.
4 Aiding re-expansion of lung tissue.
5 Mobilising the thoracic cage.

Practice

The necessity for frequent and regular practice must be emphasised to all patients being taught breathing exercises. Efficient progress will not be made if the patient only does his exercises when the physiotherapist is present.

DIAPHRAGMATIC BREATHING

The term 'diaphragmatic breathing' is misleading since the diaphragm also plays an important part in lower thoracic expansion. Perhaps breathing control by correct use of the diaphragm would more accurately describe the following technique, but throughout the text 'diaphragmatic breathing' is used for want of a more concise term. The uses of diaphragmatic breathing are:
1 To minimise the work of breathing.
2 To help control breathing during attacks of dyspnoea and during exertion.
3 To improve ventilation of the bases of the lungs.

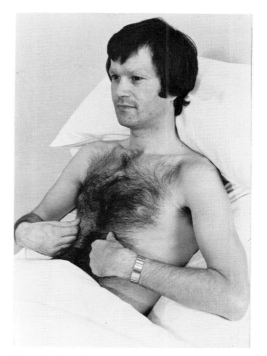

Fig. 8. *Diaphragmatic breathing.*

To teach diaphragmatic breathing the patient should be positioned so that his back and head are fully supported and his abdominal wall relaxed. If he is in bed, he should sit as high as possible with his knees slightly bent, or if he is out of bed, a high backed chair without arms is most suitable. The physiotherapist's hands rest lightly on the anterior costal margins to stimulate and palpate the movement occurring; later the patient is instructed to feel the movement himself (fig. 8).

He breathes out as quietly as possible,

13

while relaxing the shoulders and chest and sinking the lower ribs down and in towards the mid-line. He is then told to breathe in gently and to 'feel the air coming in round his waist'. The upper chest and shoulders remain relaxed throughout. The emphasis is on gentle breathing with the minimum of effort. The patient should breathe at his own rate and no attempt should be made to slow this down until controlled diaphragmatic breathing is achieved. Breathing through the nose is preferable in order to warm, moisten and filter the air, but when breathless it is often easier to breathe in and out through the mouth. The patient is closely observed during the training period so that the following common faults may be avoided:

1 *Forced expiration.* During controlled diaphragmatic breathing expiration must be completely passive; it is vital to remember that any forcing or prolongation of expiration will tend to increase airways obstruction.[1,2] In normal expiration the airways shorten and become narrower; therefore if the airways are already partially obstructed and the patient forces expiration, the flow of air will be further impeded. Forced expiration produces a rise in intrapleural pressure; air trapping may result if damaged collapsible airways are compressed by a rise in intrapleural pressure. Forced expiration (huffing) is of value in assisting the removal of secretions in both medical and surgical patients (p. 19) but should be avoided during attempts at breathing control.

2 *Prolonged expiration.* Patients should not be encouraged to attempt to empty their lungs to the residual capacity. Respiration which follows will be irregular and inefficient. The pattern tends to revert to uncontrolled upper chest breathing with the accessory muscles of respiration coming into action.

3 *Trick movements* of the abdomen. The abdominal musculature may be contracted and relaxed without any resultant effect on ventilation.

4 *Over use of the upper chest* and accessory muscles is discouraged, as this can inhibit movement of the diaphragm and increase the oxygen consumption due to the extra muscle work incurred.

THORACIC EXPANSION EXERCISES

It is unlikely that localised breathing exercises help ventilate isolated lobes of the lung, but they are useful for improving movement of the thoracic cage and for assisting the removal of secretions. These exercises have for many years been referred to as 'localised expansion exercises', but as they are used to emphasise movement of the thoracic cage rather than the underlying lobes of the lungs, the name 'thoracic expansion exercises' seems more suitable.

Pressure is applied to appropriate areas of the chest wall; utilising proprioceptive stimuli more effective movement of these areas is obtained. An active inspiration is followed by a relaxed expiration. The patient should be in a half-lying position with the knees slightly flexed over a pillow, or where possible sitting on an upright chair or stool. The physiotherapist should position herself so that she can compare the movement of the two sides of the chest. Later, some of these exercises can be practised sitting in front of a mirror.

Thoracic expansion exercises are useful in conjunction with postural drainage. While appropriately positioned the exercises may be carried out with percussion or self percussion (p 20.).

14

(a)   Unilateral lower thoracic expansion

Unilateral lower thoracic expansion is thought to make use of the 'bucket handle' movement of the ribs, thus increasing the contraction of the outer fibres of the diaphragm.

The physiotherapist places the palm of her hand well round to the side in the mid-axillary line over the 7th, 8th and 9th ribs. The patient should be instructed to relax and breathe out, and feel the lower ribs sinking down and in; this movement should not be forced. At the end of expiration, the physiotherapist should apply firm pressure to the area described. The patient should be instructed with the next inspiration to expand the lower ribs against her hand. The pressure should not be excessive, as this could restrict rather than assist the move-ment. At full inspiration the pressure is released and not reapplied until just before the patient is ready to breathe in again.

When the patient understands the localised movement required, he is taught to apply the pressure himself. This can be done in one of the following ways:

1   With the palm of the hand placed well back in the mid-axillary line (fig. 9). If wrist extension is limited this method is unsuitable.
2   With the back of the fingers; the wrist being held in the mid-position or slight flexion.
3   With the palm of the opposite hand (fig. 10).

Any simulation of costal expansion by side-flexion of the spine should be recognised and corrected and the patient should not be allowed to elevate his shoulder girdle when positioning his hands.

Many patients with obstructive airways

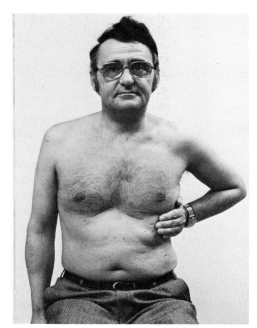

Fig. 9. *Unilateral lower thoracic expansion.*

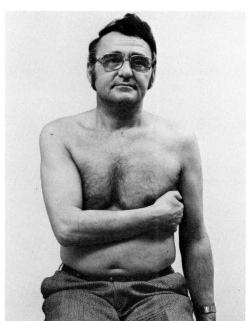

Fig. 10. *Unilateral lower thoracic expansion.*

disease must first achieve quiet expiration with relaxation of the over-inflated thoracic cage before they attempt basal expansion. The emphasis in surgical patients should be on the inspiratory phase; holding the maximum inspiration for one or two seconds is helpful. This will assist aeration of the peripheral alveoli by promoting the expansion of areas of poor compliance.

(b) Bilateral lower thoracic expansion

Bilateral lower thoracic expansion exercises can be a useful progression of treatment for post-operative patients.

Pressure is applied in the mid-axillary line to both sides of the lower chest with the palms or backs of the hands. The technique

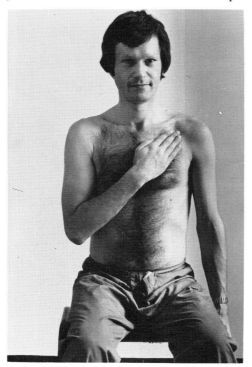

Fig. 11. *Apical expansion.*

used is the same as for unilateral expansion.

It is not advisable to use this exercise for the 'upper chest breather', particularly if the patient is applying his own pressure, as it is difficult to relax the shoulder girdle adequately.

(c) Apical expansion (fig. 11)

This is useful when there is restricted upper chest movement, e.g. following gross pleural effusion (p. 61) or incomplete expansion of lung tissue, particularly where there is an apical pneumothorax, e.g. following lobectomy.

Pressure is applied below the clavicle using the tips of the fingers. The patient breathes in, expanding the chest forwards and upwards against the pressure of the fingers. The shoulders should be relaxed and the expansion held momentarily before expiration. If the patient finds this exercise difficult he is instructed to hold his breath for a moment on full inspiration and then to sniff two or three times before breathing out.

(d) Posterior lower thoracic expansion

When movement is restricted in this area this exercise can be useful.

The patient should sit leaning forward from the hips with a straight back. Pressure is given unilaterally over the posterior aspect of the lower ribs and he can be taught to give this pressure himself.

BELT EXERCISES FOR THORACIC EXPANSION

It may be helpful for the patient to apply his own resistance, using a belt. By this method it is possible to relax the shoulder girdle more effectively, and many patients practise more conscientiously when a piece of equipment is involved.

Upholstery webbing makes suitable belts for this purpose. The width should be 5–7 cm (2–2½ in) and the length about 2 metres (6 feet) according to the patient's size.

The patient should be seated on a stool or upright chair and it is often helpful to use a mirror.

(a) Unilateral lower thoracic expansion (fig. 12)

For the left side: the belt is placed round the lower chest at the level of the xiphisternum, with a short piece round the left side and held in front with the right hand. The right forearm should be pronated and the wrist in the mid-line so that the arm is in a relaxed position. The other end is crossed over the

thighs and fixed under the left thigh. At the end of the breath out the patient pulls the belt firmly; he then breathes in and expands the left side of the chest outwards against the resistance of the belt. At full inspiration the pressure is released and expansion is maintained for a moment before expiration.

The procedure is reversed for the right side.

(b) Posterior lower thoracic expansion (fig. 13)

The patient should sit leaning forward from the hips with a straight back. For the left side: the belt is placed round the back of the chest at the level of the xiphisternum. The piece of belt coming round from the left side is held forwards with the right hand in order to give pressure to the posterior

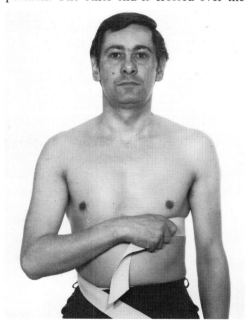

Fig. 12. *Unilateral lower thoracic expansion with belt.*

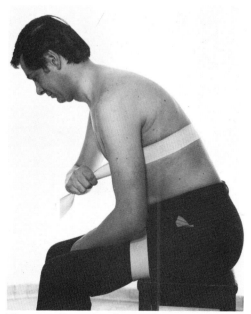

Fig. 13. *Posterior lower thoracic expansion with belt.*

17

part of the ribs. The other end of the belt is crossed over the thighs and is fixed under the left thigh. At the end of the breath out the patient pulls the belt firmly forwards and he then breathes in and expands the ribs backwards against the resistance of the belt. At full inspiration the pressure is released and expansion is maintained for a moment before expiration.

The procedure is reversed for the right side.

POSTURAL DRAINAGE

The patient is positioned to allow gravity to assist the drainage of secretions from specific areas of the lungs. The positions are based on the anatomy of the bronchial tree as shown in the diagrams (fig. 14). The value of postural drainage in the clearance of excess bronchial secretions has been established.[3,4]

Appropriate positioning should be accom-

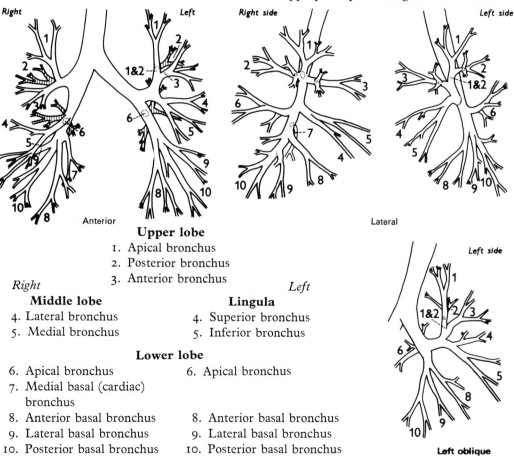

Upper lobe
1. Apical bronchus
2. Posterior bronchus
3. Anterior bronchus

Right

Middle lobe	*Left* **Lingula**
4. Lateral bronchus	4. Superior bronchus
5. Medial bronchus	5. Inferior bronchus

Lower lobe
6. Apical bronchus	6. Apical bronchus
7. Medial basal (cardiac) bronchus	
8. Anterior basal bronchus	8. Anterior basal bronchus
9. Lateral basal bronchus	9. Lateral basal bronchus
10. Posterior basal bronchus	10. Posterior basal bronchus

Fig. 14. *Diagram illustrating the bronchopulmonary nomenclature approved by the Thoracic Society. Reproduced by permission of the Editors of* Thorax.

18

panied by active participation and requires the patient's full concentration. The treatment is ineffective if the patient lies passively in a postural drainage position.

The techniques available to assist clearance of bronchial secretions are:

1 *Thoracic expansion exercises* (p. 14)
The increase in the length and diameter of the airways above that of normal tidal volume, may loosen or dislodge bronchial secretions.

2 *Forced expiratory manoeuvre—cough or huff*
A forced expiratory manoeuvre produces compression and narrowing within the airways from a point dependent on lung volume.[5] At high lung volumes this point lies in the trachea and main bronchi. Under normal circumstances bronchial secretions are effectively cleared from this region by coughing or huffing at high lung volumes. As the lung volume decreases, the point at which this dynamic compression[6] takes place moves further down the bronchial tree and is accompanied by a rapid vibratory movement of the wall. Progressively deeper portions of the airways can therefore be cleared. In the absence of chest disease the narrowing is evenly distributed, but in patients with airways obstruction it may be more marked and unevenly distributed.

To produce a cough, a forced expiratory effort is made against a closed glottis causing a rise in intrathoracic pressure. The glottis then opens abruptly so that a large pressure gradient exists between the alveolar pressure and the upper tracheal pressure (now atmospheric). A very rapid flow results.

The high intrathoracic pressure inverts the posterior membrane of the intrathoracic trachea and narrows it to one-sixth of its normal area (figs. 15 and 16). The rapid flow combined with this narrowing increases the explosive force of the air which dislodges mucus and foreign particles, bringing them to the pharynx.

To produce a huff, a forced expiratory effort is made, but the glottis remains open and the intrathoracic pressure does not rise to such high levels. The intrathoracic pressure generated, again compresses and narrows the intrathoracic trachea and bronchi and an increased expiratory flow is achieved. Mucus and foreign particles are dislodged and moved up the bronchial tree.

The use of the forced expiration technique in conjunction with postural drainage has been shown to increase the efficiency of clearance of secretions without increasing bronchospasm.[7,8] The forced expiration technique consists of one or two huffs

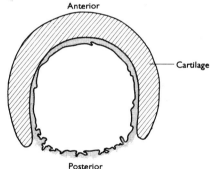

Fig. 15. *Trachea during normal breathing.*

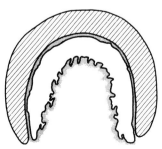

Fig. 16. *Trachea during cough—internal area reduced to $\frac{1}{6}$ of its normal area.*

(forced expirations) from mid lung volume to low lung volume, followed by a period of relaxed diaphragmatic breathing. When the secretions reach the large airways, they are cleared by a huff or cough at high lung volume. To prevent the occurrence of bronchospasm or to avoid increase in bronchospasm if it is already present, a period of diaphragmatic breathing is essential (fig. 17).

It has been shown that the mean maximum transpulmonary pressure during voluntary coughing is greater than during forced expiration.[9] A cough in patients with airways obstruction therefore produces greater compression and narrowing of the airways than a huff. This sudden airway collapse limits flow and reduces the efficiency of the cough in bronchial clearance. This,

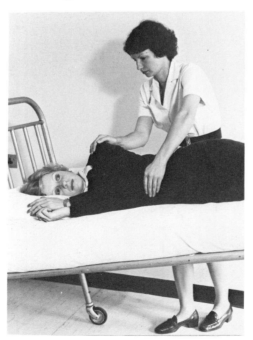

Fig. 17. *Diaphragmatic breathing. By courtesy of* Physiotherapy (1979) **65,** 304.

combined with clinical observations that a series of coughs without intervening inspirations is more exhausting than a single continuous huff down to the same lung volume is further evidence to support the use of the huff.

In attempting to clear secretions from the small airways, a huff started at mid lung volume and continued down to low lung volume is the most efficient. After taking a short breath in, the patient breathes out forcefully through the mouth, contracting the abdominal muscles at the same time. Breathing out loudly with a partially closed larynx or just clearing the back of the throat does not produce an effective huff. Children as young as three years old can be taught to huff, but may need to practise by blowing through a tube.[10]

To produce an effective cough it is important to take a deep breath before coughing and to contract the abdominal muscles during the cough. After two or three coughs another deep breath should be taken; the patient should not be allowed to go into an uncontrolled paroxysm of coughing as this is exhausting. If the patient persists in coughing without breathing in, cough syncope occasionally occurs. As with huffing, relaxed diaphragmatic breathing should be interspersed between short bouts of coughing.

It has been shown that the efficacy of the cough is improved by stabilising the trachea with the neck extended in some patients and in others with the neck flexed.[11]

3 Percussion

Clapping of the chest wall produces an energy wave which is transmitted through the chest wall to the airways. This mechanical effect is thought to loosen mucus from the bronchial walls and appears to be more effective when combined with thoracic expansion exercises than with breathing at normal tidal volume.

Clapping is carried out with the hands slightly cupped and by quick, relaxed flexion and extension of the wrists (fig. 18). It should be performed over clothes or a blanket as it is not intended to stimulate the skin. Many patients are able to do self-percussion (fig. 19).

There are several mechanical percussors available, but there is no evidence at present to suggest that bronchial secretions are cleared more efficiently when using one of these devices.

In the adolescent and adult patient with cystic fibrosis carrying out his own treatment, it has been shown that a mechanical percussor gives no additional benefit if postural drainage is combined with the forced expiration technique.[12]

4   Vibratory chest shaking

Mechanical energy is again transmitted through the chest wall. The manoeuvre is performed only during the expiratory phase of breathing and therefore has the added effect of increasing the expiratory flow rate.

Relaxed hands are placed on the appropriate area of the thorax and by using her body weight the physiotherapist produces a vibratory shaking of the chest wall during expiration. Shaking reinforces the effect of the forced expiration technique in clearing bronchial secretions. Many patients are able to assist their own postural drainage by giving compression over the lateral aspect of the chest wall.[13] A brisk adduction movement of the upper arm from an angle of about 45° abduction, is combined with the forced expiration (fig. 20). Self-compression over the anterior segments of the upper

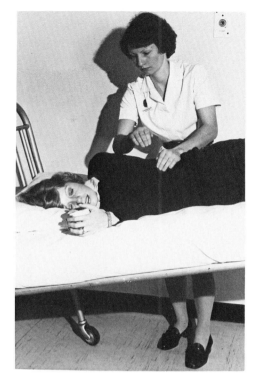

Fig. 18. *Percussion.*

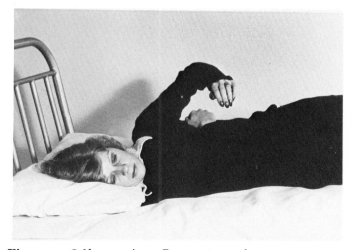

Fig. 19. *Self-percussion. By courtesy of* Physiotherapy (1979) **65**, 304.

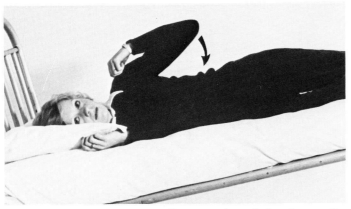

Fig. 20. *Self-compression of the chest wall.*
By courtesy of Physiotherapy (1979) **65,** 304.

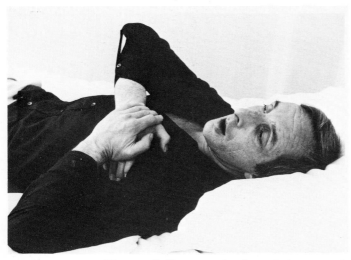

Fig. 21. *Self-compression for anterior segment of the left upper lobe.*

lobes can be used when draining these areas (fig. 21). On completion of a period of postural drainage, self-compression can be useful in the sitting position. Both arms are adducted firmly in conjunction with a forced expiration (fig. 22). Instruction in self-compression should be omitted until the patient has perfected his huffing technique.

Treatment programme for postural drainage

Each appropriate postural drainage position should ideally be maintained until the affected area is clear of secretions. The length of time required varies with each individual, but with active treatment an area is usually cleared in 10–20 minutes. Postural drainage may be required 1–6 times a day according to the patient's condition. If several areas of the lung are affected, it may not be possible to drain all of them in one session. Different areas can be drained at different times.

Many patients like to have a programme outlined for the postural drainage session. While the physiotherapist is with the patient she will give assistance, but if she leaves the patient at intervals he should continue the active treatment.

The programme must be adapted to each individual's requirements but an example could be:

(a) 3 or 4 thoracic expansion exercises, combined with percussion (by an assistant or the patient himself)

(b) pause for relaxed diaphragmatic breathing

(c) 1 or 2 huffs from mid lung volume to low lung volume, combined with chest shaking (by an assistant, or self-compression)

(d) pause for controlled breathing

When secretions reach the upper airways another huff or cough is added, followed by diaphragmatic breathing before returning to the expansion exercises. This cycle is repeated until the area being drained is clear.

To complete the treatment the patient can sit on the edge of the bed, or on a chair and clear any remaining secretions from the upper airways by using the huff with or without chest compression (fig. 22).

It is inadvisable to carry out postural drainage immediately after a meal, as the patient may tend to feel nauseated or even vomit and will not perform the treatment adequately. Postural drainage is also unsuitable immediately before a meal because the patient may have become too exhausted to enjoy his food. Some patients find it easier to cough productively after having a warm drink.

Postural drainage at home

Many patients who require postural drainage at home are able to carry out their treatment independently and efficiently using the forced expiration technique. Others who are more disabled will benefit from percussion and chest shaking given by an assistant in conjunction with the forced expiration technique. When teaching relatives or friends how to percuss and shake, it is essential that they understand the necessity for the periods of relaxed diaphragmatic breathing.

Patients who are too frail to manage chest compression and have no one to assist at home are able to move secretions by effective huffing. The vibratory action of the posterior membrane of the trachea and main bronchi in addition to the dynamic compression of the airways during the forced expiratory manoeuvre promotes movement of the secretions.

The postural drainage positions where the patient is lying prone make self-percussion and chest compression difficult, but independent treatment can be successful by means of breathing exercises and the forced expiration technique.

A patient who is in hospital and who needs to continue postural drainage at home, often benefits from carrying out his own treatment

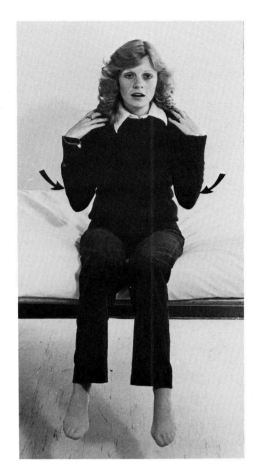

Fig. 22. *Self-compression, sitting. By courtesy of* Physiotherapy (1979) **65**, 304.

for one or two days prior to discharge. The physiotherapist, having carefully instructed the patient, supervises the treatment during these last days. By this means the patient gains the confidence required to know that he can manage without help at home. The areas requiring drainage and the time needed for treatment must be discussed with each patient. In most cases treatment will be required for at least 15–20 minutes twice daily.

The means of positioning the patient at home must be established. It is difficult for the majority of patients to elevate the foot of the bed at home. Some patients have a bed in a spare room that they keep in a tipped position. Others have a frame to tilt the whole body to a suitable angle (fig. 55 and 56). A simple, but less comfortable, method is to place a sprung sofa cushion or a 15 cm (6 in) pile of newspapers or magazines, tied tightly together, in the centre of the bed with two or three pillows on top (fig. 23). The patient can lie over this in varying positions to drain several areas of the lungs. Alternatively, a firm wedge of polyether foam can be obtained, but this is only suitable for children and light adults.

These simple methods may not provide an efficient angle of tip for some patients suffering from severe basal bronchiectasis or cystic fibrosis. It may be necessary to arrange for the loan of a frame or hospital tipping bed. The deep tipping position that is sometimes used with the patients lying over the side of the bed is unsuitable. Most patients find it uncomfortable and it mainly drains the posterior basal segments of the lower lobes.

Small children and infants can be given postural drainage by placing them over the knee (fig. 24). It is usually most convenient

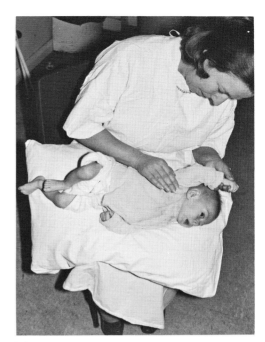

Fig. 24. *Postural drainage for a baby. By permission of Cystic Fibrosis Research Trust.*

to give this treatment immediately prior to a feed.

Modified postural drainage

Some patients suffer from orthopnoea and cannot lie flat without becoming dyspnoeic. If a patient has secretions at the lung bases and is likely to become distressed by orthodox postural drainage, it is better to compromise and position him in a high side-lying position or as flat as possible on alternate sides, without tipping the foot of the bed. In this position thoracic expansion and the forced expiration technique combined with percussion and shaking can be given as usual. If this position does not cause distress, the foot of the bed can be elevated slightly at the next treatment.

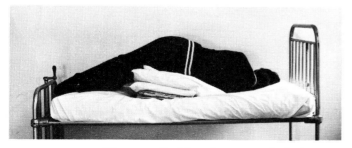

Fig. 23. *Position for postural drainage at home.*

24

Adjuncts to postural drainage

Bronchodilators. If a bronchodilator has been prescribed, this should be used before postural drainage.

Humidification. When secretions are tenacious, or airways plugged, additional high humidity is helpful preceding postural drainage. This can be administered by means of a humidifier or nebuliser containing sterile water or normal saline (p. 106).

IPPB. Patients with tenacious secretions and poor chest movement who have not responded to the treatments described, or those who become exhausted even during short treatments, may benefit by using IPPB in conjunction with postural drainage (p. 95).

Contra-indications to postural drainage, percussion and shaking

Conditions that contra-indicate postural drainage include recent haemoptysis, severe hypertension, cerebral oedema, aortic and cerebral aneurysms, many cardiac conditions where arrhythmias or pulmonary oedema are present and conditions of the oesophagus or diaphragm causing regurgitation of the gastric contents. In many cases of acute asthma and severe emphysema, dyspnoea would be increased by postural drainage for the lung bases and a modified position is used.

Neither percussion nor chest shaking are painful procedures if they are carried out skilfully. Obviously the pressure exerted on the thorax must be modified according to the build of the patient as well as the chest condition. A patient with osteoporosis or metastatic deposits affecting the ribs or vertebral column must be treated with great care.

Other contra-indications to percussion and shaking include haemoptysis, acute pleuritic pain and active pulmonary tuberculosis. Provided that breathing exercises, the forced expiration technique and coughing are carried out effectively, percussion and vibrations are rarely indicated for adults following cardiothoracic surgery. If a patient is nursed on a ventilator, vibrations or chest shaking may be required (p. 88).

Bronchography

If there appears to be an excessive quantity of secretions which could prevent adequate outlining of the bronchi by the contrast medium in a bronchogram, the patient should be given appropriate postural drainage before the procedure.

After a bronchogram the majority of the contrast medium is sucked into the peripheral bronchi during inspiration, and is gradually absorbed into the blood stream. The contrast medium remaining in the upper airways is removed by the action of the cilia and effective huffing and coughing. Although postural drainage is not essential for a patient with normal airways, a brief session with assistance from a physiotherapist immediately following the procedure makes the patient more comfortable.

Postural drainage is required for those patients with bronchiectasis. The contrast medium is unlikely to be sucked as far into the periphery because of the blockage of the small airways by sputum and endobronchial disease. The cilia are usually destroyed in these bronchiectatic airways and postural drainage speeds up the procedure of clearing the contrast medium from the bronchi.

It is important that patients have nothing to eat or drink for at least three hours after a bronchogram, until the effect of the local anaesthetic has worn off.

If the bronchogram has been performed through the cricothyroid membrane, the patient is instructed to give pressure with a finger over the cricothyroid cartilage whenever he huffs or coughs, for at least six hours after the procedure, to avoid subcutaneous (surgical) emphysema.

Postural drainage positions (figs. 25–35)

LOBE			POSTURE
Upper Lobe	**1.**	Apical bronchus	**1.** Sitting upright; with slight variations according to the position of the lesion, i.e. slightly leaning backwards, forwards or sideways.
	2.	Posterior bronchus (a) Right	**2a.** Lying on the left side horizontally, and then turned 45° on to the face, resting against a pillow, with another supporting the head.
		(b) Left	**2b.** Lying on the right side turned 45° on to the face, with 3 pillows arranged to lift the shoulders 30 cm (12 in) from the bed.
	3.	Anterior bronchus	**3.** Lying supine with the knees slightly flexed.
Middle Lobe	**4.**	Lateral bronchus	**4 & 5.** Lying supine with the body a quarter turned to the left maintained by a pillow under the right side from shoulder to hip. Foot of the bed raised 35 cm (14 in): chest tilted to an angle of 15°.
	5.	Medial bronchus	
Lingula	**4.**	Superior bronchus	**4 & 5.** Lying supine with the body a quarter turned to the right maintained by a pillow under the left side from shoulder to hip. Foot of the bed raised 35 cm (14 in): chest tilted to an angle of 15°.
	5.	Inferior bronchus	
Lower Lobe	**6.**	Apical bronchus	**6.** Lying prone with a pillow under the abdomen.
	7.	Medial basal (cardiac) bronchus	**7.** Lying on the right side with a pillow under the hips. Foot of the bed raised 45 cm (18 in): chest tilted to an angle of 20°.
	8.	Anterior basal bronchus	**8.** Lying supine with the buttocks resting on a pillow and the knees flexed. Foot of the bed raised 45 cm (18 in): chest tilted to an angle of 20°.
	9.	Lateral basal bronchus	**9.** Lying on the opposite side with a pillow under the hips. Foot of the bed raised 45 cm (18 in): chest tilted to an angle of 20°.
	10.	Posterior basal bronchus	**10.** Lying prone with a pillow under the hips. Foot of the bed raised 45 cm (18 in): chest tilted to an angle of 20°.

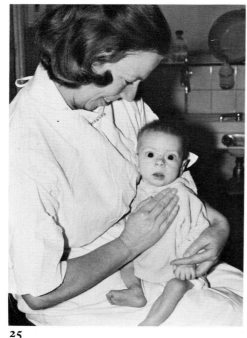

25

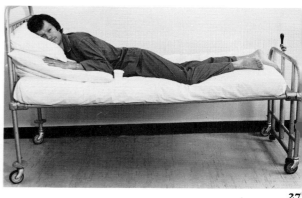

27

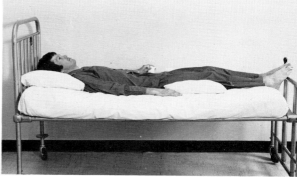

28

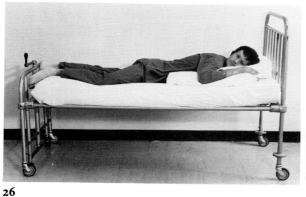

26

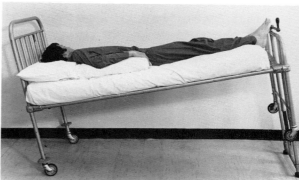

29

Fig. 25. *Apical segment, left upper lobe. By permission of Cystic Fibrosis Research Trust.*
Fig. 26. *Posterior segment, right upper lobe.*

Fig. 27. *Posterior segment, left upper lobe.*
Fig. 28. *Anterior segments, upper lobes.*
Fig. 29. *Right middle lobe.*

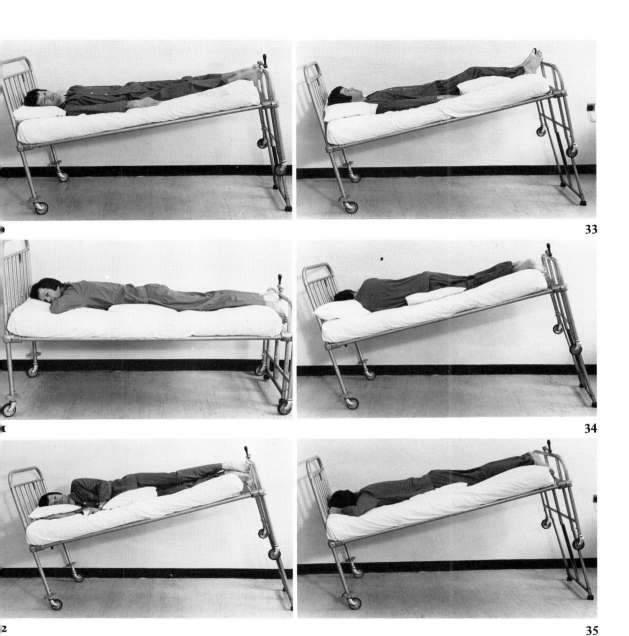

Fig. 30. *Lingula.*
Fig. 31. *Apical segments, lower lobes.*
Fig. 32. *Right medial basal and left lateral basal segments, lower lobes.*

Fig. 33. *Anterior basal segments, lower lobes.*
Fig. 34. *Lateral basal segment, right lower lobe.*
Fig. 35. *Posterior basal segments, lower lobes.*

References

1. GANDEVIA B. (1963) The spirogram of gross expiratory tracheobronchial collapse in emphysema. *Quarterly Journal of Medicine*, New Series XXXII **125**, 23.

2. DONALDSON A. & GANDEVIA B. (1962) The physiotherapy of emphysema. *Australian Journal of Physiotherapy* **8**, (2), 55.

3. COCHRANE G.M., WEBBER B.A. & CLARKE S.W. (1977). Effects of sputum on pulmonary function. *British Medical Journal* ii, 1181.

4. BATEMAN J.R.M., NEWMAN S.P., DAUNT K.M., PAVIA D. & CLARKE S.W. (1979) Regional lung clearance of excessive bronchial secretions during chest physiotherapy in patients with stable chronic airways obstruction. *Lancet* i, 294.

5. MEAD J., TURNER J.M., MACKLEM P.T. & LITTLE J.B. (1967) Significance of the relationship between lung recoil and maximum expiratory flow. *Journal of Applied Physiology* **22**, (1), 95.

6. DE KOCK M.A. (1977) *Dynamic Bronchoscopy*. Springer-Verlag, Berlin.

7. PRYOR J.A., WEBBER B.A., HODSON M.E. & BATTEN J.C. (1979) Evaluation of the forced expiration technique as an adjunct to postural drainage in treatment of cystic fibrosis. *British Medical Journal* ii, 417.

8. PRYOR J.A. & WEBBER B.A. (1979). An evaluation of the forced expiration technique as an adjunct to postural drainage. *Physiotherapy* **65**, (10), 304. *Erratum:* p. 304, col. 2, lines 6 and 7. '. . . combined with chest compression, performed by the patient alone' *should read* '. . . combined with chest shaking and percussion by the physiotherapist.'

9. LANGLANDS J. (1967). The dynamics of cough in health and in chronic bronchitis. *Thorax* **22**, 88.

10. THOMPSON B.J. (1978) *Asthma and your child*. 5th new revised edition. Pegasus Press, Christchurch, New Zealand.

11. RUNNALS M.J. (1980) Coughing and the chronic obstructive airways disease patient. *Proceedings of the 8th International Congress of the World Confederation of Physical Therapy, Israel (1978)* 129.

12. PRYOR J.A., PARKER R.A. & WEBBER B.A. (1980) A comparison of mechanical and manual percussion as adjuncts to postural drainage in the treatment of cystic fibrosis in adolescents and adults. *Physiotherapy* (in press).

13. THOMPSON B.J. (1980) *Better breathing*. 4th new revised edition. Pegasus Press, Christchurch, New Zealand.

5 Oxygen therapy

Oxygen therapy is often required in the management of patients with chest disease, but it is important to control the concentration of oxygen in some clinical circumstances.

An understanding of when oxygen must be prescribed with caution requires some knowledge of the normal chemical control of breathing.

In health, the level of the arterial carbon dioxide tension is the most important single factor controlling the rate and depth of breathing. A variety of mechanisms stimulate breathing when metabolic requirements are increased, as for example during exercise, and the level of carbon dioxide in the arterial blood remains surprisingly constant. An increase in this level beyond the normal range causes a sensation of severe breathlessness and stimulates the healthy person to hyperventilate vigorously, so removing the excess carbon dioxide and restoring the level to normal.

Some chronic lung diseases are characterised by the patient's tendency to breathe inadequately because the work of breathing is excessive and the efficiency of gas exchange is lowered by airway obstruction. A good example of such a condition is chronic bronchitis with secondary emphysema. If breathing is inadequate, the level of carbon dioxide in the blood tends to rise and the level of oxygen tends to fall. The respiratory centre slowly becomes acclimatised to the abnormally high level of carbon dioxide in the arterial blood and no longer responds by stimulating an increase in the rate and depth of breathing. When the respiratory centre no longer matches respiratory effort to the patient's requirements, the only stimulus which keeps the patient breathing regularly is the lack of oxygen (hypoxia) in the blood.

Hypoxia is dangerous because many organs, e.g. the heart and kidneys, suffer from oxygen lack. If hypoxia is relieved by the administration of high concentrations of oxygen, the last effective stimulus to respiration is removed and breathing becomes progressively more shallow and ineffective, so allowing the carbon dioxide level to rise even further. The elevated carbon dioxide level, hypercapnia, renders the patient drowsy and unco-operative and eventually comatose. He is unable to cough and secretions accumulate in the lungs so adding to his respiratory disability. The oxygen lack has been relieved so he retains a 'good' colour, and often looks unusually flushed and hot because of the effects of excess carbon dioxide on the skin. This condition is very dangerous and may be fatal.

Controlled oxygen therapy, the administration of *low* concentrations of oxygen (24–35%) will *partly* relieve the hypoxia, so reducing the risk of damage to the body, without completely eliminating the stimulus to breathe. The level of carbon dioxide may rise a little when even low concentrations of oxygen are used, but in many patients it is possible to reach an equilibrium position in which both carbon dioxide and oxygen levels in the blood are acceptable. This is best achieved by serial measurement of blood gas values; alternatively, the oxygen concentration may be increased *slowly* (over several hours) up to 28%, observing the patient for any deterioration in conscious level or ability to cough and co-operate. Any deterioration in the mental state indicates that excessive oxygen has been used and the concentration must be readjusted. If a satisfactory position cannot be achieved or if serious hypoxia persists in spite of all attempts to remove secretions and relieve spasm, intubation and intermittent positive pressure ventilation (IPPV) are generally necessary.

Not all patients with chronic lung disease respond in this way. In acute asthma, the patient may even breathe more deeply or frequently than is necessary to maintain the normal level of carbon dioxide in the blood, in an attempt to relieve the hypoxia which is always a common feature of the condition.

In the older age groups, or those with chronic asthma, and in all patients when fatigued, this ability to hyperventilate is lost and inadequate ventilation and elevation of the carbon dioxide level in the blood may follow. Until this stage is reached, most patients with asthma benefit from oxygen in high concentrations.

In another group of disorders (pulmonary oedema, fibrosing alveolitis, sarcoidosis and pulmonary embolism) the ability to absorb oxygen is impaired to a much greater degree than the ability to excrete carbon dioxide, largely because a considerable percentage of the pulmonary blood flows to parts of the lung which are not being properly ventilated and the 'good' areas of lung compensate for the 'bad' in terms of carbon dioxide removal but not for the uptake of oxygen. This is because of the different diffusing capacities of carbon dioxide and oxygen. These patients are always very breathless. They generally breathe more deeply and frequently than is necessary to maintain a normal carbon dioxide level, in an attempt to relieve the hypoxia. They require oxygen in the highest possible concentration and there is no risk of respiratory depression because the respiratory centre never loses its normal sensitivity to carbon dioxide.

A variety of masks is available to provide oxygen therapy. The masks which operate on the venturi principle provide a controlled percentage of oxygen by entraining air and humidity from the surrounding atmosphere. Additional humidification can be obtained by an adapter fitted over the air-entraining holes and connected by wide bore tubing to a humidifier (p. 108).

Nasal cannulae and masks which do not utilise the venturi principle deliver dry oxygen unless some form of humidification is placed in the circuit. Compressed oxygen

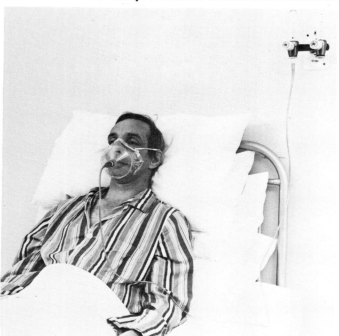

Fig. 36. *Venturi mask for oxygen therapy.*

bubbled through water obtains some moisture, but much of this is lost by condensation in narrow bore tubing before it reaches the patient. To provide more effective humidification, wide bore tubing must connect the oxygen mask to a humidifier.

If a patient is receiving oxygen therapy, the mask should not be removed during breathing exercises or postural drainage except for expectoration.

Oxygen may be used to drive an intermittent positive pressure breathing apparatus for treatment in conjunction with physiotherapy. With many of these machines, the percentage of oxygen received by the patient will be considerably higher than the controlled percentage delivered by the appropriate venturi mask (fig. 36), e.g. in the treatment of the chronic bronchitic. This higher percentage is rarely dangerous during treatment, because the patient's ventilation is assisted and the removal of secretions from the chest as a result of treatment often leads to an improvement in the general condition. It has been suggested that a few patients become more drowsy during or after IPPB treatment because of the high percentage of oxygen received. A study has shown that increased drowsiness (caused by hypercapnia) can occur whether oxygen or air is used to power the IPPB device and that this deterioration is not dependent on the driving gas but on inappropriate setting of the ventilator. The pressure and flow controls must be set to provide an adequate tidal volume, particular attention being required when treating patients with a rigid thoracic cage.[1]

When treating patients with severe hypoxia, e.g. in acute asthma, fibrosing alveolitis or left ventricular failure, oxygen is required and it is dangerous to use an IPPB machine driven entirely by compressed air. Thus IPPB should be powered either by compressed oxygen with the air entrainment device in use, or by compressed air with an attachment to provide a controlled, optimal, concentration of added oxygen.

When inhaling drugs from a nebuliser, without IPPB, the patient is breathing spontaneously. A high concentration of oxygen to power the nebuliser could be dangerous in the case of a hypercapnic patient and the nebuliser should be powered by air (p. 103).

It is important to remember that oxygen is a drug and must, like all drugs, be carefully used so that undesirable side-effects may be avoided.

Reference

1. STARKE I.D., WEBBER B.A. & BRANTHWAITE M.A. (1979) IPPB and hypercapnia in respiratory failure: The effect of different concentrations of inspired oxygen on arterial blood gas tensions. *Anaesthesia* **34,** 283.

6 Medical conditions

TYPES OF DISABILITY

Two disorders characterise many medical chest diseases. Although these features are combined in many conditions, one of them usually predominates. The disorders are as follows:

1 Obstructive airways disease

The flow of air through the lungs may be reduced by obstruction in the airways. It can be assessed by measuring the FEV$_1$ (forced expiratory volume in 1 second) which is normally 70-80% of the FVC (forced vital capacity). The FVC and FEV$_1$ are recorded on machines which give a spirogram trace, such as the Vitalograph (fig. 37). Alternatively, the Peak Expiratory Flow Rate may be measured by means of the Wright Peak Flow Meter or the Mini-Wright Peak Flow Meter. These devices measure maximum

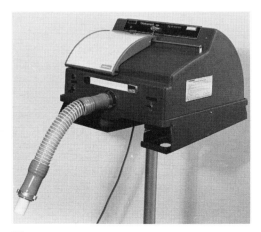

Fig. 37. *The Vitalograph.*

flow over 10 milli-seconds at the beginning of expiration (figs. 38 and 39).

If the FEV$_1$ and PEFR improve following the administration of a bronchodilator the condition is recognised as *reversible airways obstruction* (fig. 40); this is frequently seen in asthma and chronic bronchitis. Reversible airways obstruction is caused by bronchospasm, oedema of the bronchial mucosa or excessive secretions; a combination of all three is often present.

If the FEV$_1$ and PEFR do not improve following administration of a bronchodilator, this is known as *irreversible airways obstruction*. It is a sign of structural damage of the airways and is seen in emphysema, severe chronic bronchitis and generalised bronchiectasis.

The patient may feel some relief after a bronchodilator, and this may be due to very slight reversibility in the airways obstruction which is shown by increase in FVC, although no change is registered in PEFR or FEV$_1$. This increase in FVC reflects the fact that some deflation of the overdistended lungs has occurred as a result of slight dilatation of the airways.

The Peak Flow Meter and Mini-Wright Peak Flow Meter are simple, portable devices, useful to assess airways obstruction where there is a considerable degree of reversibility, but with largely irreversible airways disease where minimal change in the airways is important, spirometry is more informative.

A patient's response to bronchodilator drugs can be accurately assessed by measurements of FEV$_1$ and FVC. Bronchodilator drugs should not have been given for at least six hours preceding the test. Stable baseline readings, with correct technique, must first be obtained. The best result of two or three attempts is taken, allowing at least a thirty second pause between them. Baseline readings are repeated at five minute intervals until the maximum pre-treatment level is known. Some patients will continue to improve over several minutes while others will soon reach a plateau or decrease their FEV_1 or FVC.

The bronchodilator is then inhaled and spirometry is repeated at the appropriate time interval for the particular drug. After salbutamol (Ventolin), or terbutaline (Bricanyl), readings can be made at 15- and 30-minute intervals, whereas with the slower acting atropine methonitrate and its derivatives, recordings are made 40 and 60 minutes from the time of inhalation. In each case recordings should be continued until the maximum response is achieved, for example if the response to salbutamol is greater at 30 minutes than at 15 minutes, the spirometry is repeated at 10-minute intervals until a plateau or fall in FEV_1 or FVC is recorded.

This principle can be applied when comparing different methods of delivery of the same drug or when comparing the response to two different bronchodilators. If comparing the response of a patient to Ventolin by pressurised aerosol and a nebulised solution of Ventolin, measurements are made until maximum response is reached after inhalation by pressurised aerosol and then the nebulised solution is given immediately. Any additional response is determind by the post-nebuliser recordings. If response to one method of delivery is determined on one occasion and to the other method on a separate occasion, it is impossible to compare the results accurately because the baseline readings and other factors such as the time of testing and the dose of steroid drugs may be different.

Similarly when comparing the response to two different drugs (e.g. salbutamol and atropine) the second should be given as soon

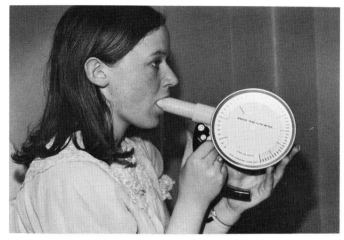

Fig. 38. *Wright Peak Flow Meter in use.*

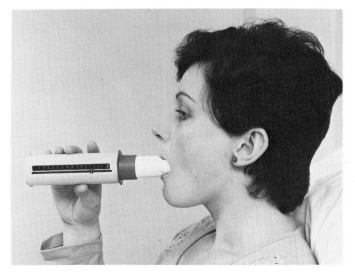

Fig. 39. *Mini-Wright Peak Flow Meter.*

35

as maximum response has been achieved with the first.

2   Restrictive pulmonary disease

Pulmonary expansion may be restricted by abnormalities of the rib cage, pleura or lungs.

Disorders of the rib cage include conditions such as ankylosing spondylitis and kypho-scoliosis. The flow of air in the lungs is reduced although there is no bronchial disease.

With disorders of the pleura or lungs, such as pleural fibrosis, interstitial pulmonary fibrosis (fibrosing alveolitis), or pulmonary oedema, there is a decrease in pulmonary compliance (increased stiffness) which restricts lung expansion.

The lung volumes are reduced in patients with restrictive lung disease and to achieve adequate gaseous exchange breathing may be rapid (tachypnoea).

Diseases of the lung itself often interfere with the alveolar wall adding difficulties of gas transfer to those of pulmonary restriction.

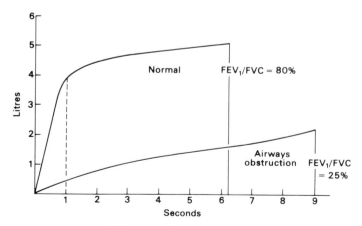

Fig. 40. *Spirometry.* FEV$_1$ *in normal and obstructed airways. By courtesy of Dr D.A.Ryland.*

ASSESSMENT OF THE PATIENT

Before starting treatment, the physiotherapist should assess the condition of the patient. Important facts are ascertained by reading the medical history, looking at chest radiographs and their reports, as well as reports of relevant investigations such as lung function tests, blood gases and bacteriology.

Brief clinical examination of the patient, observation and simple questioning will provide further information. The following are some questions that the physiotherapist should consider:

1   Relevant *history* of the illness.

2   *Exercise tolerance:* is the patient short of breath (dyspnoeic) at rest, or only on exertion? Has it prevented him from working? How far can he walk in 12 minutes? (p. 43).

3   *Breathing pattern:* is the thorax held in an overinflated position? Are the accessory muscles of respiration being used? Is there any deformity or obvious restriction of movement? When a deep breath is taken, is there a sudden 'catch' in breathing due to pleuritic pain? Is there equal expansion of both sides of the lower rib cage? Chest measurements can be taken if no other means of assessment is available, but cannot be reproduced with accuracy. They are taken at full inspiration, full expiration and in the resting position, at three levels:

(a)   in the axilla at the level of the 4th rib

(b)   in the epigastric region at the level of the 9th costal cartilage

(c)   in the subcostal region with the tape measure below the ribs.

4   *Breath sounds:* auscultation is helpful if the physiotherapist is familiar with the use of a stethoscope, but valuable information such as the presence of wheeze, stridor, or

moist sounds can be acquired by listening to the patient's breathing and coughing without a stethoscope.

5   *Cough:* is the cough productive?

6   *Sputum:* what volume is produced daily? Is it mucoid (clear or white), mucopurulent, purulent (infected), rusty (typical of lobar pneumonia), blood stained, or does it contain plugs or casts (typical of some cases of asthma and bronchopulmonary aspergillosis (p. 59)?

7   *Chest pain:* is there pain due to the pulmonary condition such as pleuritic pain? Is there skeletal pain due to osteoporosis or metastatic disease? Is it due to myocardial insufficiency?

8   *Colour:* is the patient cyanosed?

9   *Airways obstruction:* in obstructive airways disease what are the FEV$_1$ and FVC, or PEFR? Where simple lung function tests have previously been recorded, repeating the tests will enable comparisons to be made giving an indication of the severity and nature of the condition. This also provides an assessment of the degree of reversibility which may be expected as a result of treatment.

OBSTRUCTIVE AIRWAYS DISEASES

This group of diseases includes chronic bronchitis, emphysema and asthma.

CHRONIC BRONCHITIS AND EMPHYSEMA

Chronic bronchitis has been defined[1] as a condition in which there is a chronic or recurrent increase above the normal in the volume of bronchial mucous secretion, sufficient to cause expectoration, when this condition is not due to localised broncho-pulmonary disease. The words 'chronic' or 'recurrent' may be further defined as when the cough is present on most days during at least three months in each of two successive years.

A later definition[2] subdivided chronic bronchitis into simple chronic bronchitis, chronic or recurrent mucopurulent bronchitis and chronic obstructive bronchitis.

Emphysema is a condition in which there is increase beyond the normal in the size of air spaces distal to the terminal bronchiole, with destructive changes in their walls.[1]

These conditions previously described in this way are currently under review,[3] but in simple terms a patient with chronic bronchitis and emphysema has irreversible airways obstruction with chronic productive cough. Recent work has shown that there are two distinct disorders, obstructive and hypersecretory, which commonly occur together, but may develop independently.[3] With the hypersecretory disorder there is hypertrophy of the mucus-secreting glands in the bronchial walls and an increase in goblet cells in the epithelial lining of the bronchial tree causing expectoration and a predisposition to bronchial infection. The obstructive disorder causes impairment of expiratory flow leading to eventual disability.

Many patients have a combination of these disorders and repeated infections may damage the alveoli with acute inflammation and their weakened walls may rupture. The bronchioles become scarred and distorted, so that on expiration air trapping occurs. Cigarette smoking is a major factor in the development of both the hypersecretory and obstructive disorders and patients should be urged to stop.

If hypersecretion alone is present there will be chronic productive cough without noticeable dyspnoea. There are usually no radiological changes of emphysema and the diffusing capacity of the lungs is normal. In the more advanced stage of the disease hypercapnia (a raised $Pa\text{CO}_2$) is common, the patient is cyanosed and cor pulmonale develops. These patients are sometimes known as 'blue bloaters'.

The signs and symptoms of those patients with predominantly an obstructive disorder are dyspnoea, usually with wheeze, a reduced FEV$_1$ with little or no response to a bronchodilator showing that there is largely irreversible airways obstruction. With progression of the disease the patient becomes breathless at rest, uses the accessory muscles of respiration and develops over inflation of the upper chest with paradoxical indrawing of the lower rib cage on inspiration owing to the pull of the low flattened diaphragm. When radiological evidence of emphysema is present there will be a low flattened diaphragm, a large retrosternal air space and the heart may appear as a narrow vertical shadow. Bullae may be visible. In addition to a severe obstructive defect, pulmonary function tests show an increase in total lung capacity and residual volume and the ratio of the residual volume to total lung capacity is raised indicating air trapping. The diffusing capacity of the lungs is impaired. These patients, sometimes known as 'pink puffers', maintain a normal or low level of arterial carbon dioxide by hyperventilating in an effort to obtain an adequate arterial oxygen level. Cardiac failure does not develop until the terminal stage of the disease.

Many patients have both the hypersecretory and obstructive disorders in varying proportions leading to a mixture of the signs and symptoms.

A minority of patients with emphysema may have the condition known as 'primary emphysema' which develops without any previous history of chest disease and is commonly associated with a familial deficiency in alpha$_1$-antitrypsin. Sputum production is unusual in these cases unless there is superimposed infection. The alveolar walls may disintegrate over a relatively short period leading to terminal respiratory failure.

Aims of treatment

1 To remove excess bronchial secretions and reduce airways obstruction.
2 To reduce the work of breathing.
3 To teach control of breathing.
4 To mobilise the thorax.
5 To increase the patient's exercise tolerance.

1 Removal of excess bronchial secretions and reduction of airways obstruction

All patients with chronic bronchitis should carry out regular postural drainage during the productive phases of their disease (see postural drainage at home, p. oo). In the absence of infection the secretions are mucoid. Mucoid secretions are often small in volume but clearance may require considerable effort on the part of the patient. Purulent secretions, associated with infection, tend to be larger in volume, but the patient may be able to expectorate more easily.

In patients with 'primary emphysema', secretions are usually absent, but during an infective episode sputum may be present and postural drainage is indicated. In some patients with chronic bronchitis where emphysema is predominant, tipping may aggravate dyspnoea and postural drainage may need to be modified (p. 24).

Chest shaking should not be over-vigorous if the patient has been on high maintenance doses of corticosteroids as there is a tendency to osteoporosis and rib or vertebral fractures may result.

If the patient is unable to clear his chest adequately, it may be helpful to provide increased ventilation and humidification by means of intermittent positive pressure breathing (IPPB). This, in conjunction with postural drainage, will facilitate expectoration (p. 95).

There is often an element of bronchospasm associated with these diseases. If reversible bronchospasm is present, a bronchodilator may be given prior to postural drainage with IPPB, a nebuliser (p. 104) or a pressurised aerosol (p. 48). IPPB should not be used in the presence of emphysematous bullae because of the risk of causing a pneumothorax. Vitalograph recordings before and after inhalation of a bronchodilator will indicate the degree of reversibility in the airways (p. 34).

Some patients with obstructive airways disease demonstrate a bronchodilator response to salbutamol. Atropine has been shown to benefit some patients who do not respond to salbutamol alone and others demonstrate reversibility to salbutamol and atropine given together.[1]

2   Breathing control and reduction of the work of breathing

During an attack of dyspnoea, the patient with bronchitis and/or emphysema tends to hold his chest in a position of inspiration. There is overactivity of the accessory muscles, and diaphragmatic movement is inhibited. In severe emphysema there is often paradoxical movement of the chest wall, the lower ribs being drawn in on inspiration.

The pattern of breathing developed by an emphysematous patient is a short uncontrolled inspiration, using the accessory muscles, followed by a prolonged and often forced expiration. This forced expiration produces a rise in intrathoracic pressure which may cause closure of the airways that are either damaged, or no longer have the support of normal elastic lung tissue (fig. 41). This uncontrolled pattern of breathing is an exhausting and uneconomical method of ventilation, which the physiotherapist should attempt to reverse.

Some emphysematous patients spontaneously develop a technique of 'pursed-lip' breathing. Such patients breathe out through the mouth with the lips held together loosely in a pursed position. It is

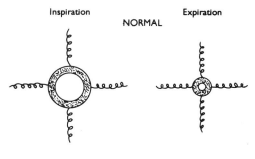

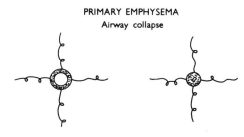

Fig. 41. *Airway collapse. By courtesy of Professor Lynne Reid.*

possible that this improves respiration by increasing the end expiratory pressure in a manner similar to the effect used in artificial ventilation. This method of breathing should not be discouraged, provided that it is carried out correctly in a relaxed manner. If an attempt is made to teach this form of breathing to a patient who has not developed it spontaneously, there is a great danger of expiration becoming forced, thus defeating the purpose of the technique. Unless this pattern is already established, it should be omitted from the treatment programme.

All patients with obstructive airways disease are taught to breathe with an active inspiratory phase using the diaphragm and a passive relaxed expiratory phase. If the patient can control his breathing, it can be of great benefit during attacks of dyspnoea. The rest positions (figs. 42–47) encourage maximal relaxation of the upper chest and freedom of movement of the lower chest. They can be adapted to different situations in everyday life. At this stage the rate of breathing is not important, but control of the upper chest is essential. The patient may

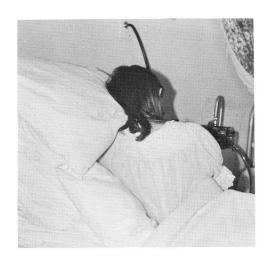

Fig. 43. *High side-lying (posterior aspect).*

prefer to breathe with his mouth open during an attack of dyspnoea. He should be encouraged to breathe gently with the lower chest without prolonging expiration (p. 14). When control of breathing has been achieved an effort should be made to slow down the respiratory rate. In some severely emphysematous patients it may be impossible to eliminate the use of the accessory muscles of respiration completely.

HIGH SIDE-LYING (figs. 42 and 43)

The patient lies on one side, slightly rolled forward, with a slope of three or four pillows to raise the shoulders, and an extra pillow placed to fill the gap between the waist and axilla to prevent him sliding down the bed and to maintain a straight thoracic spine. The top pillow should be above the shoulder supporting only the head and neck. The underneath forearm can be placed either under the head pillow or resting on the bed under the pillow at the waist. The knees are slightly bent and the top leg placed in front of the lower one. This position is helpful for

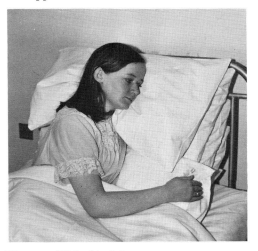

Fig. 42. *High side-lying.*

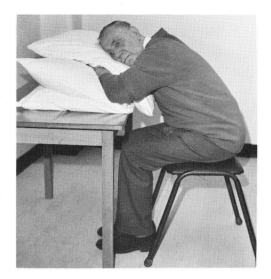

Fig. 44. *Forward lean sitting.*

patients in acute respiratory distress, or at night for those suffering from orthopnoea.

FORWARD LEAN SITTING (fig. 44)

Many patients find this position comfortable. Two or three pillows are placed on a table and the patient can relax with the upper chest and head resting against them. The patient should maintain a straight thoracic and lumbar spine to avoid inhibiting diaphragmatic movement.

RELAXED SITTING (fig. 45)

This is a useful position and can be taken up unobtrusively in public places. Many patients are inclined to grip their knees and raise their shoulders when in distress, but if they can sit leaning forward with the fore-arms resting on the thighs and the wrists relaxed, they will recover more quickly. If

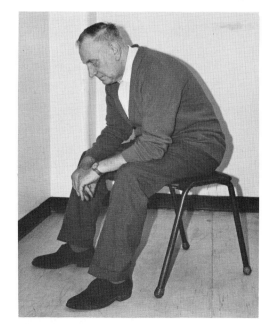

Fig. 45. *Relaxed sitting.*

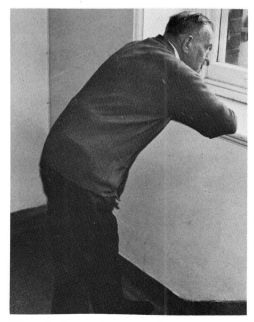

Fig. 46. *Forward lean standing.*

there is still a tendency to put pressure on the hands and forearms, some patients find relaxation easier with the forearms supinated and palms upwards. Care must be taken to ensure that the lumbar spine is not flexed, as this could impede free forward movement of the abdominal wall.

FORWARD LEAN STANDING (fig. 46)

If there is nowhere to sit, distressed patients are inclined to grasp the nearest available object and hold themselves in a tense position. They should be encouraged to lean forward with the forearms resting on an object of suitable height.

RELAXED STANDING (fig. 47)

The distressed patient may also gain relief by leaning back against the wall or an upright support. The feet should be approximately 30 centimetres from the wall, the shoulders relaxed and arms hanging by the sides.

CONTROL OF BREATHING
DURING EXERCISE

When the patient is able to control his breathing in these relaxed positions he should practise while sitting and standing upright without support. Progression can then be made to control of breathing while walking on the level, on stairs and on hills. Many patients tend to hold their breath during exercise. Breathing in rhythm with their steps can be helpful; for example, breathing out for two steps and in for one step, out for one step and in for one step or out for three steps and in for two steps. A breathing pattern must be established for each individual.

Some patients tend to become distressed

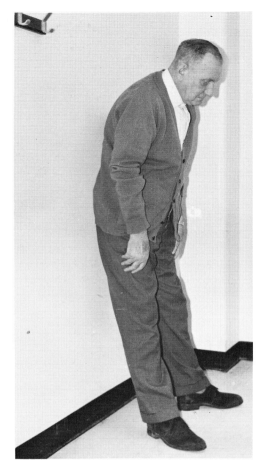

Fig. 47. *Relaxed standing.*

when bending forward (e.g. to tie shoe laces). Many of them breathe in before bending down and experience discomfort due to the upward pressure of the abdominal contents against the flattened diaphragm. This discomfort is less if breathing out is encouraged whilst bending down; breathing in takes place during the return to an upright position.

Although pulmonary function tests do not show any significant improvement in patients who have been taught controlled breathing,[5] they appear to derive benefit from the fact that they are breathing in a more economical manner. By eliminating unnecessary muscular activity during respiration, the work of breathing is reduced.

3 Mobilisation of the thorax

Treatment is not progressed until the patient has mastered breathing control and relaxation of the upper chest both during and between attacks of dyspnoea.

Thoracic expansion exercises (p. 14) are then started. In the patients where severe chest deformity has not developed, belt exercises may be useful. By improving the mobility of the lower thoracic cage together with relaxation of the upper chest, the patient should achieve a more normal pattern of breathing.

In patients with emphysema, the domes of the diaphragm are flattened or even inverted. This abnormal position of the diaphragm can cause rib retraction on inspiration, but with perseverance a little lateral basal movement may eventually be achieved.[6]

4 Increase of exercise tolerance

At one time it was common practice in physiotherapy departments to hold breathing classes for groups of patients, but it is now generally accepted that adults benefit more from individual treatment.

The aim of physiotherapy for severely disabled patients is to increase their exercise tolerance to enable them to carry out useful daily activities. Patients should be encouraged to be as mobile and active as possible. Their exercise tolerance may be increased by gradually increasing the distances walked, both on the level and on slopes and stairs, while practising breathing control.

The 12-minute walking test is a simple and reproducible method of assessing the exercise ability of the chronic breathless patient. It is described[7] as the greatest distance that the subject can walk in 12 minutes in a level enclosed corridor, regardless of whether or not he has to stop for rest. At least one practice 12-minute walk is necessary before the results are reproducible. If the practice test is carried out within a day or two of the next test there is no need to do more than one practice, but if a longer period elapses two practice walks are necessary as shown in a study where walks were performed at monthly intervals.[8] The test is helpful in assessment before beginning an exercise programme and to determine progress.

A simple graduated exercise scheme has been shown to increase exercise tolerance as judged by the 12-minute walking test, while ventilatory function tests remained unchanged.[9] An exercise scheme designed by McGavin et al.[10] for patients to carry out at home, starts with the daily climbing of 5 steps for 2 minutes and week by week the number of steps or minutes is gradually increased. The aim is to build up to climbing 10 steps for 10 minutes at least once daily. If no staircase is available, a similar scheme can be devised walking on the level.

There are differing views on the physiological changes in heart rate and oxygen uptake produced by exercise training of the chronic bronchitic,[9] but the most likely physiological explanation for improvement concerns the oxygen cost of exercise. With training the activity is performed more efficiently and requires less oxygen. There is also a psychological component in improved exercise tolerance. Fear is reduced once the patient is persuaded that breathlessness is not harmful. Training helps him to gain confidence and often increases tolerance to the sensation of breathlessness.

In some hospitals a graduated training programme using a treadmill or bicycle ergometer is used, but it seems more appropriate to provide a programme that can be carried out in the home and has the effect of training for an activity related to daily life.

Inhalation of a bronchodilator preceding exercise can improve exercise tolerance, although the extent of the improvement does not correlate with changes in FEV_1 or FVC.[11]

A few patients are so handicapped that they may need portable oxygen therapy and in some cases the assistance of a high walking frame to enable them to get about (fig. 48).

Home instruction

It is essential that all patients with chronic obstructive airways disease continue physiotherapy at home. Prolonged out-patient treatment is unnecessary if careful instructions have been given.

Acute exacerbation of chronic bronchitis

If a patient with chronic bronchitis develops an acute infection, his condition may deteriorate rapidly. Excess bronchial secretion is produced and although some is expectorated, a considerable quantity remains in the bronchial tree contributing to airways obstruction. Swelling of the bronchial mucosa due to the infection will decrease the lumen of the air passages and further contribute to obstruction. This obstruction to ventilation results in inadequate gas exchange in the periphery of the lung: the Po_2 (oxygen tension) of the arterial blood falls, while the Pco_2 (carbon dioxide tension) of the arterial blood rises. As a result, the patient becomes drowsy and confused and his breathing becomes erratic, shallow and inefficient.

At this stage, vigorous physiotherapy is essential. The usual methods of postural drainage may not be effective because the patient may be unable to co-operate with breathing exercises and coughing. IPPB can be of great value here, and may obviate the need for intubation (p. 95 for techniques with IPPB). Assisted ventilation with vigor-

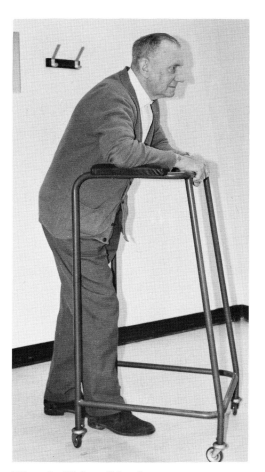

Fig. 48. *High walking frame.*

ous chest shaking and postural drainage, as tolerated, aerate the lungs more effectively and loosen secretions. The patient often begins to cough spontaneously and becomes more alert. During the early, acute stage of the exacerbation, it may be necessary to repeat the treatment at hourly intervals.

Dehydration is often a problem in the acute stage making expectoration of viscid secretions difficult. Encouraging the patient to take frequent drinks will help, together with humidification of the inspired gases. A venturi mask providing controlled oxygen therapy is usually required and to humidify such a mask adequately, a humidity adapter is useful (p. 108).

Cor pulmonale

Cor pulmonale has been defined[1] as: 'Hypertrophy of the right ventricle resulting from diseases affecting the function and/or structure of the lung, except when these pulmonary alterations are the result of diseases that primarily affect the left side of the heart or of congenital heart disease.'

Cor pulmonale most commonly occurs in association with long-standing pulmonary disease such as chronic bronchitis or bronchiectasis. It is also seen in patients with kypho-scoliosis. It rarely occurs in primary emphysema.

A respiratory infection superimposed on one of these conditions frequently precipitates cor pulmonale. The respiratory infection causes carbon dioxide retention and hypoxia and these together cause constriction of the pulmonary arterioles so producing pulmonary hypertension. Many pulmonary blood vessels are obliterated by disease of lung tissue, thus making the passage of blood through the pulmonary circulation even more difficult. A radiograph of the chest will show cardiac enlargement and dilatation of the main pulmonary arteries. In the later stages of cor pulmonale, right ventricular failure develops due to the enormous work load and continuing hypoxia.

Physiotherapy is required to clear excess secretions and to improve alveolar ventilation. Other treatment includes oxygen therapy, antibiotics and diuretics. It must be understood that the right-sided heart failure in cor pulmonale will not be relieved until the chest condition has been treated. Physiotherapy, therefore, is of prime importance.

ASTHMA

Asthma is defined as narrowing of the airways which varies over short periods of time either spontaneously or as a result of treatment.

Asthmatic patients may be classified as being atopic or non-atopic. Atopic subjects have elevated serum levels of total IgE antibody, with specific IgE antibody to allergens such as grass pollen and house dust mite and have positive immediate skin prick test reactions elicited by such allergens. Symptoms often start in infancy with flexural eczema, followed by rhinitis and asthma provoked by exposure to specific allergens. There is often also a family history of eczema, hay fever and asthma.

IgE antibody fixes to mast cells in the skin, eyes, nose and airways. Reaction of IgE on the surface of the mast cell with specific antigen such as grass pollen, leads to the release of mediators, such as histamine, from the cell which cause local swelling in the skin (weal and flare reaction) and smooth muscle contraction (narrowing of the airways).

Non-atopic subjects do not have elevated total IgE levels in their serum. Skin tests with allergens such as grass pollen and house dust mite are negative and no specific IgE antibody to such allergens is found in their serum. Their asthma generally starts in adult life. They have not usually had eczema or hay fever and do not generally give a family history of these, although they may have a family history of asthma.

Both atopics and non-atopics may have asthmatic reactions provoked by other agents, both specific and non-specific. Such specific agents include occupational agents (such as toluene di-isocyanate and platinum salts) and drugs (such as aspirin and propranolol). Non-specific factors provoking asthma include upper respiratory tract infections, emotinal upsets, exercise and inhalation of cold air.

Where provoking factors can be identified in either atopic or non-atopic individuals there is the possibility of finding effective treatment whether by removing the cause (occupational agent or known allergen), desensitising the patient, or giving an appropriate prophylactic drug such as Intal (sodium cromoglycate) prior to exercise or exposure to the provoking stimulus.

Patients with intermittent asthmatic attacks will probably require regular bronchodilators and Intal, and those with persistent airway narrowing may also require long-term inhaled or oral corticosteroid treatment.

The narrowing of the airways in asthma is caused by a combination of three factors: bronchospasm (smooth muscle contraction), oedema of the mucous membrane and plugging with tenacious exudate. On admission to hospital with an acute, severe attack of asthma, the patient is likely to be in respiratory distress using the accessory muscles of respiration. Wheeze is often audible, but in very severe cases there may be no wheeze, due to lack of respiratory reserve. Wheeze, or lack of wheeze, is therefore not a satisfactory indication of severity of acute asthma.

Assessment of the severity of an attack is made by measurement of airways obstruction (FEV_1 or PEFR), arterial blood gas levels, pulse rate and the degree of arterial paradox (pulsus paradoxus). As airways obstruction increases, the arterial carbon dioxide level at first falls, but may gradually rise as the patient becomes exhausted. The arterial oxygen level although low, is of less value in assessing the severity of asthma. Tachycardia is a feature of acute severe asthma. There may be a marked degree of arterial paradox which reflects abnormal intrathoracic pressures produced by airways obstruction. Normally there is a fall in systolic blood pressure of up to 10 mmHg during inspiration, but levels of up to 40 mmHg may be present in a severe asthmatic attack. Increasing asthma also affects the electrocardiograph recording and changes suggesting acute pulmonary hypertension may be seen.

Drug and oxygen therapy are instituted immediately after assessment of the patient. The drugs commonly used are an intravenous infusion of aminophylline and hydrocortisone, with the addition of inhaled salbutamol and oral corticosteroids. Physiotherapy is usually requested soon after admission to hospital.

In rare cases where drug therapy is not controlling the asthmatic attack, in that the FEV_1 is not improving and the arterial carbon dioxide level is rising as the patient becomes more exhausted, intubation and ventilation may be indicated (p. 91).

Physiotherapists treat patients with a widely varying degree of asthma, ranging from those with a severe attack to those who are almost symptom free.

Aims of physiotherapy

1   To relieve bronchospasm.
2   To encourage relaxation and gain control of breathing.
3   To assist removal of secretions.
4   To improve the pattern of breathing.

1   Relief of bronchospasm

This is the most important aspect of the treatment as it will be impossible to mobilise the secretions until bronchodilatation has started. The physiotherapist should remember that coughing and postural drainage if inappropriately used may aggravate bronchospasm.

Administration of a bronchodilator by means of IPPB is often very effective during the acute stage. When IPPB is used correctly, it appears to reduce the work of breathing, at the same time as delivering the drug (p. 95). The patient should be in a comfortable position, either in high side-lying (p. 40), or sitting upright well supported by pillows. IPPB with the prescribed bronchodilator is given and the patient encouraged to relax the upper chest and shoulder girdle. Treatment may be repeated 4 hourly during the acute stage, and gradually reduced as the patient improves. Patients who on awakening demonstrate a persistent fall in peak expiratory flow rate, should not have the early morning treatment withdrawn until their condition stabilises.

Simple lung function tests are carried out before and after treatment to assess the response to the bronchodilator (p. 34). A peak flow chart provides a useful record of the condition of asthmatic patients. On the

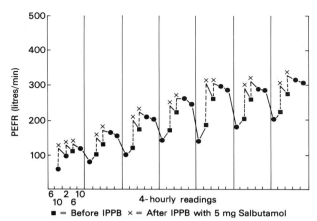

Fig. 49. *Peak flow chart. By courtesy of Physiotherapy* (1976) **62,** 57.

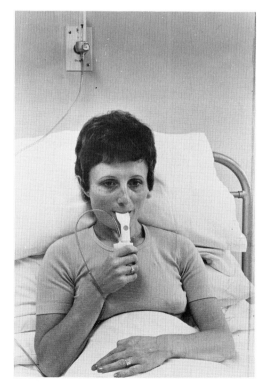

Fig. 50. *Inhalation from a nebuliser.*

chart shown (fig. 49) 4 hourly recordings have been made by the nursing staff from 6.0 a.m. to 10.0 p.m. and the physiotherapist has recorded the peak flow rate before and 15 minutes after the completion of inhalation of a bronchodilator.

When no longer in the acute stage, or if IPPB equipment is not available, the patient can inhale the bronchodilator solution from a simple nebuliser by mouthpiece (p. 104) (fig. 50). The patient should be well supported in a relaxed position and inhale using diaphragmatic breathing. It has been shown that during the recovery stage the bronchodilator response is as good using a simple nebuliser as it is with IPPB.[12] Children may be frightened by IPPB, but frequently respond well to a nebuliser.

The dosage of bronchodilator solution often prescribed in the treatment of asthma is 5 mg salbutamol (1 ml of 0·5% Ventolin respirator solution). When the patient starts to respond to other medical treatment a 2·5 mg dose is usually equally effective. Terbutaline has a similar action, the dose being 7·5 mg or 5 mg (0·75 or 0·5 ml of 1% Bricanyl respirator solution). The main side effect of these drugs is muscular tremor, especially of the hands. The physician will adjust the dosage of all bronchodilator drugs to reduce this to a minimum.

If bronchodilatation is not produced by adrenergic drugs (salbutamol, terbutaline) an anticholinergic drug, such as atropine methonitrate, may be prescribed. A dose of 3 mg (0·3 ml of 1% atropine methonitrate respirator solution) is used and maximum response may not be reached until one hour after inhalation. Common side-effects are dryness of the mouth and loss of visual accommodation. Occasionally retention of urine may occur. Although bronchial secretions are more difficult to expectorate owing to the dryness of the mouth, the viscosity of the secretions is not altered.[13] Despite these mild side-effects, atropine methonitrate has been shown to be an effective bronchodilator either alone or in combination with salbutamol.[14]

As soon as a dry pressurised aerosol such as a Ventolin inhaler produces an equally good bronchodilator response, this should be used instead of the more expensive and complicated equipment. Instruction in the correct technique for using a pressurised aerosol is often necessary and before comparative tests of bronchodilator response (p. 35) are made, it is essential to ensure that the inhaler is being used correctly.

The patient should exhale quietly and completely and having placed the aerosol up to the mouth should press it firmly whilst inhaling deeply. To be effective it is essential that the drug is released during the beginning of inspiration. After inhaling, the patient should hold his breath for a comfortable period of time before breathing out quietly through his nose.

Many patients find it easiest to use the aerosol with the lips closed round the mouthpiece, but it has been shown that better entraining of the drug is achieved with the inhaler held 4 cm away from the mouth.[15] A placebo inhaler is often helpful in teaching patients who are having difficulty in learning the technique and a modified aerosol incorporating a whistle is particularly useful.[16]

For patients who have poor co-ordination and are unable to use a pressurised aerosol effectively, the Ventolin and Becotide Rotahalers have proved invaluable. This method of delivery is also useful for children and the elderly. Another device to help those patients who have difficulty with co-ordination is the Bricanyl Spacer Inhaler.

2 Relaxation and control of breathing

Relaxation and control of breathing are important in both severe and mild asthma. The patient should be shown the relaxed positions described on p. 40–42, and encouraged to breathe gently with his diaphragm at his own rate during attacks of dyspnoea. He should only be encouraged to slow down his rate of breathing once he has gained control. With sufficient practice, breathing control in conjunction with the prescribed drugs can help during asthmatic attacks.

3 Removal of secretions

Great care must be taken not to aggravate bronchospasm when assisting with removal of secretions; if a patient is unable to expectorate, the physiotherapist should not persist with this treatment, but wait until further bronchodilatation has taken place.

As soon as coughing results in the expectoration of sputum a modified form of postural drainage (p. 24) should be started. It has been shown that the forced expiration technique does not increase bronchospasm in asthmatic patients when used to aid clearance of bronchial secretions.[17] The treatment should be given 10–15 minutes after administration of a bronchodilator. At this stage many patients start to expectorate thick, tenacious sputum which may contain casts. As the patient's condition improves, the foot of the bed can be tipped for postural drainage.

In the earlier section on relief of bronchospasm, it was stated that when an equally good response to a bronchodilator can be achieved by a nebuliser or pressurised aerosol, IPPB should be discontinued. At the stage when secretions are thick and tenacious it may be of value to continue with IPPB for the mechanical assistance in mobilising the secretions. High humidity inhaled following bronchodilators may help loosen secretions, but care must be taken to ensure that bronchospasm is not aggravated (p. 108).

Many asthmatic patients have a productive cough between attacks and should include postural drainage in their home treatment. Inhalation of a bronchodilator, if prescribed, should precede postural drainage.

4 Improvement of the breathing pattern

Lower thoracic expansion exercises should be started when there is improvement in the patient's condition. The patient should be made aware of his pattern of breathing, and should be encouraged to relax the upper chest and minimise the action of the accessory muscles. It may be helpful to practise in front of a mirror, as many patients are unaware of their faulty pattern of breathing.

Exercise for asthmatics

Exercise may induce bronchoconstriction in asthmatic patients. It has been shown that there are significantly smaller falls in FEV_1 after swimming than after running and bicycling,[18] but it is now thought that the difference is probably due to different environmental conditions. Humidification or warming of the inspired air, as in a heated swimming pool, reduces exercise-induced asthma, whereas cooler air exacerbates the asthmatic response.

Present evidence suggests that different types of exercise produce similar degrees of exercise-induced asthma provided that ventilation and the environmental conditions are similar.[19] It is thought that hyperventilation is probably the central mechanism in exercise-induced asthma, but it is not yet understood how hyperventilation and airway cooling lead to bronchoconstriction.[20]

Children with asthma often have poor posture and frequently do not participate in physical training in school. Many of them enjoy class work and often benefit from being treated in groups. It is a wise precaution to measure the FEV$_1$ or peak flow rate of these patients whenever they attend for treatment. If the readings are low, thus indicating an increase in airways obstruction, they should not join in the class and treatment should consist of administration of the prescribed

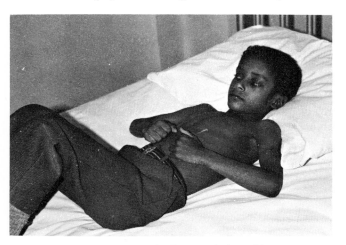

Fig. 51. *Diaphragmatic breathing.*

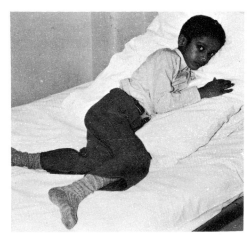

Fig. 53. *High side-lying.*

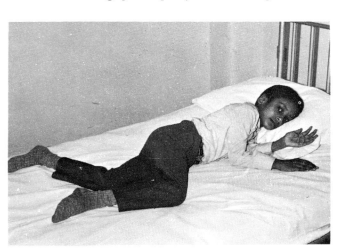

Fig. 52. *Diaphragmatic breathing in side-lying.*

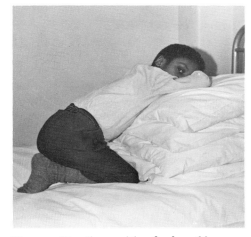

Fig. 54. *Kneeling position for breathlessness.*

50

bronchodilator followed by relaxation and breathing control and removal of secretions if present. During classes for asthmatic patients, the more vigorous exercises should not last longer than three minutes at a time and should be interspersed with relaxation and breathing control.

With improvement in drug therapy, many children with asthma are able to lead relatively normal lives, and once instruction has been given in breathing control and postural drainage, it should not be necessary to continue out-patient physiotherapy.

Bronchitis and asthma in children

Recurrent 'chestiness' in children is a very common condition. Some children even react to mild upper respiratory tract infections by coughing and wheezing, and sometimes it may be difficult to make a clear distinction between bronchitis and asthma.

Infants and children respond well to postural drainage if they have excess secretions and from the age of two or three upwards it is possible to teach elementary breathing exercises. The habit of mouth breathing should be discouraged. The principles of treatment are the same as for an adult, with modification of some positions as children are often comfortable lying flat during an attack of dyspnoea (figs. 51–54).

Instructions should be given to parents in supervision of exercises at home, and in assistance to the child during an asthma attack. Breathing exercises should be practised daily for at least ten minutes and it is often necessary to carry out postural drainage.

As children develop, the airways increase in size and the episodic narrowing of the airways may no longer be apparent.

PULMONARY INFECTIONS AND ASSOCIATED DISEASES

PNEUMONIA

Acute lobar pneumonia is not often seen in hospital since it responds quickly to antibiotic therapy if this is started in the early stages. However, from time to time cases are admitted and if physiotherapy is requested the treatment must not be confused with that appropriate for the more common bronchopneumonia.

Acute lobar pneumonia is characterised by fever, malaise and toxaemia. Pulmonary consolidation is present in one or more lobes, and it is frequently due to infection by the pneumococcus. In the early stages of the disease the patient suffers from pleuritic pain, dyspnoea and a painful cough. Pleuritic pain is an acute localised chest pain, worse on coughing or deep breathing, and is due to inflammation of the pleura overlying the consolidated lobe. The cough is usually unproductive, but there may be scanty tenacious mucoid sputum, or it may be blood stained and 'rusty' in colour. An area of consolidation will be apparent on radiography. During this stage breathing exercises are encouraged; chest shaking and percussion are not only painful, but of no benefit to the patient.

In the next stages of the disease, the pulmonary consolidation starts to resolve and as the pleuritic pain diminishes coughing becomes less painful and usually productive of mucopurulent sputum. At this stage appropriate postural drainage is instituted and assistance given to clear secretions.

Bronchopneumonia, in contrast to lobar pneumonia, is patchy in distribution and is associated primarily with bronchial inflammatory change. It is seen more frequently than lobar pneumonia and commonly in post-operative patients and in chronic bronchitics, and especially when these two situations co-exist. Physiotherapy is an essential part of the treatment regime and is instituted immediately. Purulent or muco-purulent sputum is present in considerable quantities causing obstruction of the airways. As there is no consolidation or pleural inflammation causing pleuritic pain, there is no contra-indication to early physiotherapy. This consists of breathing exercises combined with postural drainage to assist the removal of secretions. If these measures are not effective, IPPB is used to assist ventilation and clearing of secretions (p. 95).

LUNG ABSCESS

Postural drainage may be started as soon as a lung abscess is diagnosed. The abscess sometimes causes distortion of the bronchi and postural drainage positions may have to be modified to obtain effective drainage.

The use of IPPB is contra-indicated as there is a risk of causing air trapping in the cavity.

BRONCHIECTASIS

Bronchiectasis is characterised by dilatation of the bronchi associated with obstruction and infection. It can start in childhood following a respiratory infection such as pneumonia or whooping cough, or more rarely by obstruction of a bronchus as in primary tuberculosis (p. 56). Inhalation of a foreign body such as a peanut is another rare cause. Bronchiectasis occurs with cystic fibrosis, allergic bronchopulmonary asper-

gillosis (p. 59) and may complicate hypo-gammaglobulinaemia because of the patient's reduced capacity to resist bacterial infection. The diagnosis will be confirmed by a bronchogram.

Most patients have a productive cough with purulent sputum and suffer from repeated chest infections. Haemoptysis may occur in varying degrees and in some patients it may be their only symptom; this is known as 'dry' bronchiectasis.

Destruction of the cilia which are responsible for clearing the bronchi will have occurred as a result of the disease. Postural drainage is therefore essential for patients with a productive cough. Even if the cilia survive, they may beat ineffectively due to the excessive secretions. These patients will have to continue postural drainage for the rest of their lives and instruction in home management is vital.

Postural drainage is unnecessary for patients with 'dry' bronchiectasis; it may even aggravate the tendency to haemoptysis. If a mild haemoptysis occurs in productive patients, postural drainage may be continued, but percussion should be omitted for the next twenty-four hours. If severe haemoptysis occurs, physiotherapy should be discontinued temporarily until the bleeding has been controlled.

If the disease is sufficiently localised, surgery for removal of the affected lobe or lobes may be performed (p. 73).

CYSTIC FIBROSIS

Cystic fibrosis is a genetically determined disorder which has become increasingly recognised since it was first described in 1938. In this condition the exocrine glands are abnormal and the patients have an unusually high concentration of sodium in the sweat; abnormal pancreatic function and recurrent lung infections occur either together or separately. The abnormal pancreatic function results in malabsorption and steatorrhoea and the recurrent lung infections result in generalised suppurative bronchiectasis and the formation of multiple lung abscesses. The survival of these patients depends on the control of pulmonary infection and prevention of permanent lung damage. At one time it was unusual for these patients to survive over the age of 14, but with improved diagnosis and treatment many patients are now surviving to over the age of 30.

The introduction of postural drainage even before chest symptoms and signs have appeared is recommended by some physicians. This may delay the onset of chest complications and improve the overall prognosis. It should be remembered that radiological changes may be present without any detectable clinical change.

Treatment of the pulmonary complications consists of appropriate antibiotics and physiotherapy. Although antibiotic requirements may vary from time to time, physiotherapy must be a constant feature of the management even when the patient is apparently 'well'. During an exacerbation it is imperative that intensive physiotherapy is carried out. Even though the patient may attend a specialist hospital at intervals for follow up, the local hospital should be prepared to offer facilities for physiotherapy if the patient and his relatives are unable to manage at home on these occasions.

The frequency and duration of *postural drainage* must be carefully assessed for each individual and the appropriate positions taught for the affected areas of the lungs. During an exacerbation the patient may need to spend as long as 20 minutes draining each area and it is often necessary to carry out treatment six times a day. In hospital the patient can position himself early in the morning and late in the evening, or alternatively he can be positioned by the nursing staff.

Often several lobes are affected and in order to give the patient some respite, the physiotherapist may have to be satisfied with treating two or three areas at one session and the other affected areas at the next session.

The home programme must be worked out for each individual. Many patients are able to treat themselves both effectively and efficiently without assistance, if instructed in postural drainage using the forced expiration technique (p. 19). It has been shown that cystic fibrosis patients who had been relying on assistance with postural drainage at home could carry out their treatment more efficiently without assistance after being taught the forced expiration technique.[22]

A portable, but stable, tipping frame is an

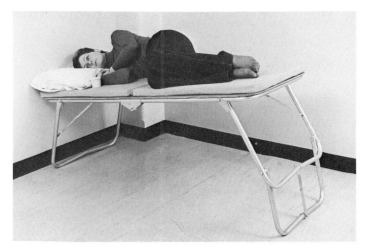

Fig. 55. *Postural drainage frame* (Chesham Engineering Ltd).

asset for many patients at home. A frame that supports the whole patient at an angle (figs. 55 and 56) is more comfortable and versatile than the frames that are angled at the centre which cannot support the patient comfortably for several of the required postural drainage positions.

Relatives of infants and small children should be instructed in the postural drainage positions appropriate for the patient and in the technique of clapping and chest shaking. It may also be necessary to instruct the relatives or friends of the adolescent and adult patient.

It is essential that the parents of the young patient realise the importance of regular treatment and encourage him to carry it out conscientiously. Postural drainage should not be given immediately following a meal. Infants should be treated just before their feeds. Patients who produce sputum only occasionally should carry out postural drainage once or twice a day. Early

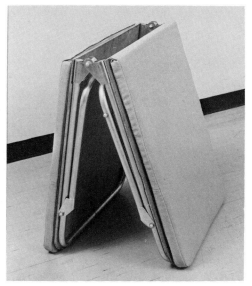

Fig. 56. *Postural drainage frame folded.*

in the morning, and/or before going to bed in the evening, are usually the most suitable times. If no specific area is apparently causing trouble, the positions for draining the lateral and posterior segments of both lower lobes are probably the most suitable to teach. If the patient has a cold, treatment must be performed more frequently until the production of excess sputum has subsided.

A physiotherapist should see the patient at regular intervals (for instance when he attends the doctor's follow-up clinic), in order to assess the chest condition, suggest any alterations in home treatment and discuss any problems that have arisen.

Difficulties are often encountered in the treatment of adolescents who become resentful of their condition and authority in general; they may rebel against any form of treatment given by their parents or doctors. It is often better for the physiotherapist to see the patient without his parents and to try to persuade him of the importance of regular drainage and to offer facilities for out-patient physiotherapy if necessary. Alternatively it is sometimes possible to teach friends how to help with postural drainage although many patients will be able to treat themselves. After the patient has left school there may be a problem of fitting in the treatment around his hours of work, but a solution must be worked out.

Breathing exercises are an integral part of the postural drainage treatment, but in addition lower thoracic expansion exercises should be practised regularly as there is a tendency to develop an over-inflated chest. Dyspnoeic patients are shown relaxation positions (p. 40) and are instructed in controlled breathing in these positions and when climbing stairs or hills.

With the development of an over-inflated

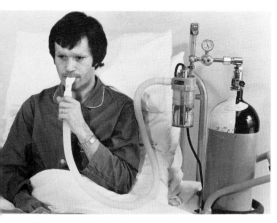

Fig. 57. *Inhalation from Puritan nebuliser.*

via a mouthpiece or mask (fig. 58). It is more effective to use a mouthpiece, with a vent for entraining additional air and for exhalation. It has been shown that with a mask many of the droplets are lost on the face and in the upper respiratory tract.[25] For small children who are unable to co-operate it may be necessary to use a

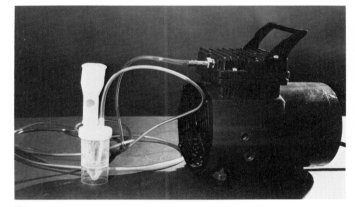

Fig. 58. *Medix Wobl Pump with Bard Inspiron Mini-Neb.*

upper chest and rigid lower rib cage, many patients tend to a kyphotic posture. Exercises to *mobilise the shoulder girdle and trunk* and to *correct posture* should be included in the treatment programme.

Participation in physical education at school should be encouraged; *general activities* such as swimming and running are also beneficial and should be continued until the patient is no longer capable of such exertion.

In some countries the regular use of *mist tents* at night has been advocated, but it has been shown that mist tent therapy evaluated over a six month period had no beneficial effect[23] and a further study has shown no decrease in sputum viscosity or enhancement of the removal of secretions.[24] During an acute exacerbation of the bronchopulmonary infection, patients often find it easier to expectorate after inhaling mist from an efficient nebuliser by mouthpiece (fig. 57). If the patient is being nursed with an oxygen mask, high humidification should be incorporated into the system with wide bore tubing (p. 108).

In this country, many patients use a small *inhalation* apparatus providing mist therapy

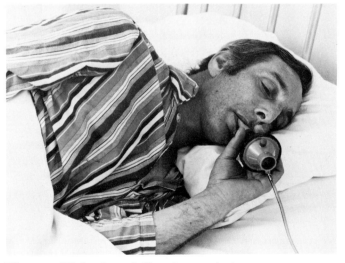

Fig. 59. *Bird micronebuliser in use during postural drainage.*

mask. The inhalation before or during postural drainage (fig. 59) helps to moisten the air passages and ease the removal of secretions. If bronchospasm is present it may be relieved by inhalation of a bronchodilator before treatment. The inhalation of an adrenergic drug such as salbutamol or terbutaline has been shown to improve cilial action.[26] Occasionally after a course of intravenous antibiotics, inhaled antibiotics may be prescribed (p. 104). The inhalation should follow postural drainage.

IPPB should be used with caution in the treatment of cystic fibrosis because there is the possibility of causing a pneumothorax and it has also been shown to increase the residual volume in these patients after a prolonged period of treatment.[27] In patients with an acute exacerbation who have become exhausted and unable to clear their secretions adequately, it has proved useful during postural drainage. Short periods of treatment, lasting a maximum of 14 days are recommended in these circumstances and the inspiratory pressure should be kept low (i.e. below 11 cmH$_2$O).

Complications of cystic fibrosis include haemoptysis and spontaneous pneumothorax. Many patients have occasional mild *haemoptyses*. If there is only slight streaking of the sputum, the postural drainage routine can be continued avoiding vigorous percussion. If a more severe haemoptysis occurs, percussion should be omitted until the bleeding decreases. Where very severe bleeding occurs, postural drainage should be temporarily discontinued, but resumed as soon as possible to remove any blood that has accumulated in the lungs.

Spontaneous pneumothorax can occur in the older patient. A small pneumothorax may absorb spontaneously and physiotherapy is continued. A larger pneumothorax may require an intercostal drainage tube, attached to an underwater seal and physiotherapy is discontinued until it has been inserted. Percussion should be avoided over the site of the tube. Analgesia may be helpful preceding treatment. Thoracic expansion exercises may be encouraged in between postural drainage sessions to assist re-expansion of the affected lung. If the air-leak persists, surgery, in the form of pleurodesis or pleurectomy, may be indicated (p. 76).

Physiotherapy should be continued during the *terminal stage* of the disease, even though it may achieve little physical improvement. Treatment will have become such an integral part of the patient's life that withdrawal at this stage would cause anxiety. The extent of treatment should be considered carefully and it should not be allowed to cause undue exhaustion. Nasopharyngeal suction should not be considered as it is an unpleasant procedure and would serve no useful purpose at this stage.

PULMONARY TUBERCULOSIS

Pulmonary tuberculosis has become less common since the improvement of public health standards and treatment by effective chemotherapy. Physiotherapy is rarely requested for this condition, but it is sometimes necessary to treat associated complications.

The first infection with the tubercle bacillus is known as *primary tuberculosis*. A small pneumonic lesion may occur in any part of the lung and the nearest lymph glands become enlarged. The lesion usually heals by fibrosis and calcification and subsequently causes no problem; occasionally it spreads through the lobe and may then cavitate. If pleural effusion occurs, thoracic expansion exercises are required (p. 14).

In infants and young children, the enlarged hilar lymph nodes may compress a bronchus and cause segmental collapse. Prolonged compression may lead to permanent bronchiectasis as in the 'middle lobe syndrome'. Another cause of segmental collapse may be discharge of caseous material from the affected lymph gland into the bronchus. Physiotherapy may be requested to attempt re-expansion of a collapsed middle lobe. The result may be disappointing but it is worth persevering with breathing exercises and postural drainage as re-expansion sometimes occurs.

Post-primary tuberculosis is a re-infection after the primary lesion. The infection usually occurs in the upper lobes or apical segments of the lower lobes. A small area of tuberculous bronchopneumonia appears at first, and this spreads by direct infection to neighbouring lung tissue. Caseation follows and the necrotic centre of the lesion is discharged into a bronchus, leaving a cavity. The patient coughs up infective sputum, some of which may be inhaled into other areas of lung, producing new tuberculous lesions. Haemoptysis occurs if there is erosion of blood vessels.

Peripheral lesions may cause pleurisy leading to tuberculous effusion or empyema. In these cases physiotherapy is important to prevent chest deformity and loss of respiratory function by pleural thickening (p. 61). There is no risk of physiotherapy causing spread of the disease once medical treatment has been established.

In contrast to acute tuberculosis with infiltration and cavitation, a chronic fibrocaseous condition may develop. Gross fibrous contraction of the upper lobes with compensatory emphysema of the lower lobes results in dyspnoea and diminished respiratory reserve. Breathing control and assistance with removal of secretions, during periods of superimposed chest infection, may be helpful. IPPB may be contra-indicated if cavitation has taken place.

A tuberculoma is a cavity with thick walls containing inspissated material which appears radiologically as a rounded opacity. It may be removed surgically since it is sometimes difficult to differentiate tuberculoma from carcinoma.

Tuberculous bronchiectasis may be a complication of either primary or post-primary tuberculosis. Postural drainage may be given, but percussion will be contra-indicated if there is a large cavity or haemoptysis. The physiotherapist should stand behind the patient when he is coughing. Treatment is carried out two or three times daily according to the quantity of sputum.

MISCELLANEOUS PULMONARY DISEASES

OCCUPATIONAL LUNG DISEASE

Several lung diseases are attributable to the inhalation of dusts, fumes or noxious substances. The most common of these 'occupational' lung diseases are coalminers' pneumoconiosis and silicosis.

Fibrotic nodules develop throughout the lungs around the particles of inhaled dust and these progress to large areas of fibrosis. The diseases may be complicated by chronic bronchitis and emphysematous changes. Symptoms include progressive dyspnoea on exertion, accompanied by cough which may be productive of mucoid sputum and recurrent exacerbations of bronchitis.

The most important aspect of management of these diseases is prevention by adequate precautions in industry and regular chest radiography for employees exposed to risk.

The aims of physiotherapy are similar to those for chronic bronchitis and emphysema: assistance with removal of secretions by postural drainage and possibly IPPB (p. 95), and instruction in breathing with economy of effort.

DIFFUSE FIBROSING ALVEOLITIS

This condition is characterised by a diffuse inflammatory process in the lung beyond the terminal bronchiole, resulting in thickening and fibrosis of the alveolar walls. This may occur rapidly in the subacute form known as the Hamman–Rich syndrome, and it may be fatal within six months. More commonly the disease progresses in the chronic form over a few years.

The characteristic symptom is progressive and unremitting dyspnoea. Pulmonary function tests show a restrictive defect with reduction in gas exchange. Radiographs show fine, diffuse mottling.

Steroids may limit the fibrosis and relieve dyspnoea in some patients. Physiotherapy is purely palliative. Instruction in breathing control may give some relief. If superimposed infections occur, IPPB and chest vibrations may assist removal of secretions.

RHEUMATOID DISEASE AND ASSOCIATED CONDITIONS

Many of the diseases allied to rheumatoid disease show respiratory manifestations and those producing symptoms may benefit from physiotherapy.

In *rheumatoid arthritis* there may be pleural effusion and pleural thickening, pulmonary nodules and diffuse interstitial fibrosis. The patient may have radiographic changes, but be asymptomatic or symptoms of dyspnoea and cough may develop. The presence of bronchopulmonary infection may be masked by anti-inflammatory drugs.

In *systemic lupus erythematosus* (SLE), pleurisy with or without an effusion often occurs accompanied by acute pleuritic pain. There may be pneumonic changes either directly due to SLE or secondary to an infection. Radiographic changes show gradual elevation of the diaphragm. This progressive lung 'shrinkage' may be caused by dysfunction of the diaphragm rather than primary pathology of the lung.[28] Lung function tests indicate a restrictive defect with reduced total lung capacity, vital capacity, lung compliance and often a reduction in diffusing capacity.

Both these conditions are treated with corticosteroids, but symptomatic treatment by the physiotherapist may be beneficial. Instruction in breathing control is given to relieve dyspnoea at rest and on exertion and thoracic expansion exercises help to maintain mobility of the thoracic cage. In cases of SLE with grossly reduced vital capacity, IPPB may assist movement of the thoracic cage or loosen secretions if they are present. In the event of an infection necessitating more vigorous physiotherapy in rheumatoid arthritis, it is advisable to consider the possibility of steroid-induced osteoporosis.

The same principles of treatment apply to other associated conditions such as systemic sclerosis (generalised scleroderma) and polyarteritis nodosa.

Ankylosing spondylitis is an acquired disease of the spine and sacroiliac joints. During the later stages of the disease the vertebral joints become immobile and the thorax becomes fixed causing a restrictive pulmonary defect.

A patient referred for physiotherapy early in the disease benefits from mobility exercises for the spine and thorax and thoracic expansion exercises to maintain movement of the rib cage. A patient whose thorax has become fixed may require assistance if he develops a bronchopulmonary infection. IPPB, with a relatively high pressure to overcome the resistance of the rib cage, may help clear bronchial secretions.

PULMONARY REACTIONS TO THE ASPERGILLUS

The aspergillus is a common fungus which causes various types of pulmonary disease. The spores of the fungus are present in the atmosphere and are particularly prevalent in Great Britain in the winter months.

In some people the aspergillus causes an immediate allergic response producing an attack of *asthma*. In these cases there is an instant positive reaction to skin testing.

In others a more complex allergic response occurs producing a disease known as *allergic bronchopulmonary aspergillosis*. Skin testing produces an immediate and a delayed response. The symptoms include inflammation and oedema of the bronchi and bronchioli which cause wheezing. Transient pulmonary infiltrates develop associated with pulmonary eosinophilia and often lead to obstruction of the bronchi and collapse of a segment or lobe. Eventually bronchiectasis may develop with fixed airways obstruction. The sputum may contain bronchial casts, often brown in colour, from which *Aspergillus fumigatus* can be cultured.

Treatment is similar to that for asthma, but whereas shaking with postural drainage may not be indicated for an asthmatic, it is always necessary in the treatment of allergic bronchopulmonary aspergillosis. Postural drainage may take longer than usual if the patient has bronchial casts, but great relief is felt once they are expectorated. IPPB with a bronchodilator preceding postural drainage is useful to relieve bronchospasm and to assist in loosening secretions. Inhalation from an ultrasonic nebuliser, or another type of efficient humidifier, preceding postural drainage often assists expectoration (p. 108).

Aspergillus fumigatus may infect cysts or cavities which have resulted from such diseases as tuberculosis, pulmonary infarction or lung abscess. An *aspergilloma* is a solid ball of fungus (mycetoma) which fills the cavity. Radiography will demonstrate a crescent of air above the opacity, which can be shown to alter position with changes of posture.

Some patients have recurrent haemoptysis while others are asymptomatic. Surgery is rarely undertaken because of the risk of spreading the fungal infection, so that an aspergilloma is often left untreated, but where haemoptyses are severe resection may be necessary.

Occasionally a patient with an aspergilloma becomes sensitive to the aspergillus in the cavity and then develops a cough, wheeze, sputum and other symptoms of allergic bronchopulmonary aspergillosis.

Inhalations of antifungal agents such as natamycin (Pimafucin) or Brilliant Green, are sometimes prescribed in the treatment of aspergilloma or allergic bronchopulmonary aspergillosis.

PULMONARY TUMOURS

Carcinoma of the bronchus is the most common tumour of the lung. The majority of these tumours arise centrally in the larger bronchi and are visible through a broncho-scope. A few develop peripherally. Histo-logically 56% are found to be squamous cell carcinoma, 37% are anaplastic (oat cell carcinoma), 6% adenocarcinoma and 1% alveolar cell carcinoma.

The first symptoms are often a dry cough and pain, but as the growth increases in size it causes progressive bronchial obstruction and production of mucopurulent sputum, leading eventually to collapse of the lung segment. Haemoptysis may result from ulceration of blood vessels and a persistent wheeze becomes apparent due to obstruction of the bronchus. Complications such as unresolved pneumonia, lung abcess or pleural effusion are not uncommon.

Surgery by lobectomy or pneumonectomy is often the treatment of choice (p. 64), but if the growth is too extensive, or too rapidly progressive (anaplastic), or the repiratory reserve is inadequate, other methods are employed.

Chemotherapy or radiotherapy may be used to produce a remission in patients unsuitable for resection, or to relieve symptoms such as obstruction of the superior vena cava. If there is infection beyond the bronchial obstruction the patient will start to expectorate purulent sputum once the tumour reduces in size. Physiotherapy by means of postural drainage and gentle vibrations can help the removal of secretions. Percussion and vigorous shaking are contra-indicated in view of possible haemoptysis or the presence of metastases in the spine or ribs.

As a result of radiotherapy, pulmonary fibrosis may develop causing dyspnoea. Instruction in breathing control, particularly when walking, is beneficial.

Physiotherapy may be requested for patients in the terminal stage of the disease to assist with removal of secretions. Postural drainage (or a modified form) with gentle vibrations may be helpful if a patient is distressed and having difficulty in clearing the airways. IPPB is contra-indicated if the tumour is partially obstructing a large bronchus as air trapping may result, but it could be used to assist clearance of bronchial secretions if the tumour is in the peripheral airways. If the patient is unable to cough and expectorate, is alert and in extreme distress, naso-tracheal suction may on rare occasions be used, but it is unjustified during the terminal stage if the patient is in a state of coma.

Adenoma and *hamartoma* are benign tumours of the lung treated by surgical removal.

PULMONARY EMBOLISM

A pulmonary embolus most commonly arises from a deep vein thrombosis in the leg or pelvis. A distinction must be drawn between massive pulmonary embolism where more than 50% of the major pulmonary artery branches are obstructed and pulmonary infarct caused by several small emboli.

Massive pulmonary embolism

A large embolus may cause sudden death. If the embolism is not immediately fatal the patient becomes suddenly shocked, dyspnoeic and complains of central chest pain. Pulmonary angiography may be used to confirm the diagnosis. Treatment may be either by intravenous anti-coagulants or emergency embolectomy. Surgery is carried out on cardiopulmonary bypass (p. 87).

Pulmonary infarction

Small emboli cause a pulmonary infarct. Diagnosis is often difficult and this serious respiratory lesion is sometimes overlooked. When the infarct extends to the lung surface, the pleura becomes involved causing acute pleuritic pain and often effusion. Haemoptysis only occurs in about 50% of cases and the source of the embolus is not always clinically detectable. Repeated small emboli may eventually lead to obstruction of the pulmonary vascular bed and cause pulmonary hypertension and right ventricular failure.

Treatment of pulmonary infarction consists of anti-coagulants, oxygen, bed rest and analgesia to relieve the pleuritic pain.

Physiotherapy is primarily prophylactic and all patients at risk are given active leg exercises and breathing exercises to assist the venous return. Patients are encouraged to carry out foot and leg exercises at frequent intervals until they are ambulant.

If a pulmonary infarct occurs, physiotherapy is discontinued until anti-coagulant therapy is established. Breathing exercises are then given to encourage movement of the affected area since chest movement is limited by the pleuritic pain. Postural drainage may assist expectoration of old blood and clot. Leg exercises are continued until the patient is ambulant.

DISEASES OF THE PLEURAL CAVITY

PLEURAL EFFUSION

Breathing exercises are important following a pleural effusion to maintain mobility of the thoracic cage before adhesions form and the pleura becomes thickened. The types of pleural effusions most commonly seen by the physiotherapist are those found in associa-tion with pneumonia, tuberculosis and trauma, and those following thoracic surgery. Pleural effusion may also be associated with cardiac failure, nephritis or intrathoracic neoplasms; these conditions do not benefit from physiotherapy.

If there is a large effusion causing dyspnoea, breathing exercises are not usually effective until the fluid has been aspirated. Thoracic expansion exercises are given to all areas of the affected side of the chest, including the apical area where there is often some flattening. Belt exercises are useful in this condition. If there is gross deformity of the chest wall, the patient is positioned lying on the unaffected side with two or three pillows under the thorax in order to open out the rib cage of the affected side. Breathing exercises are done intermittently while in this position. It may be necessary to lie in the position for twenty to thirty minutes several times a day.

EMPYEMA

Empyema, a collection of pus in the pleural cavity, is now rarely seen. It may be associated with bronchopleural fistula following pulmonary surgery. Empyema may be treated surgically by decortication (p. 77) or rib resection with insertion of a drainage tube, or medically. If patients are treated medically, by chemotherapy and possibly aspiration, thoracic expansion exercises are part of the general treatment regime. Empyema results in thickening of the pleura and restriction of lung movement. Early physiotherapy is essential so that maximum re-expansion of lung tissue and minimum permanent restriction result. Breathing exercises are necessary to prevent deformities, as with pleural effusion.

SPONTANEOUS PNEUMOTHORAX

A collection of air in the pleural cavity resulting from some pathological process, is known as spontaneous penumothorax. When the pneumothorax is small the lung often re-expands within a few days. Treatment consists of rest alone; physiotherapy is usually unnecessary. If the lung fails to re-expand, or collapses further, air must be withdrawn from the pleural cavity; an intercostal tube is inserted for a few days and the air in the pleural space withdrawn. Following the insertion of a tube, breathing exercises may be given to assist re-expansion of the lung; particular attention should be given to expansion of the apical region if there is an apical air pocket. The physiotherapist should ensure that the patient carries out a full range of movements in the shoulder joint.

In some cases the spontaneous pneumothorax recurs with consequent chest pain, dyspnoea and interference with day-to-day activities. Moreover, if any other lung disease is present such as emphysema, a recurrent pneumothorax may result in severe disability. For this reason the pleural cavity is often obliterated medically with talc or irritant oils (pleurodesis), or surgically by pleurectomy or abrasion pleurodesis (p. 77).

References

1. WORLD HEALTH ORGANIZATION (1961) Definition and diagnosis of pulmonary disease with special reference to chronic bronchitis and emphysema. *WHO Technical Report Series* **213**, 15.

2. MEDICAL RESEARCH COUNCIL (1965) Definition and classification of chronic bronchitis for clinical and epidemiological purposes. *Lancet* i, 775.

3. FLETCHER C., PETO R., TINKER C. & SPEIZER F.E. (1976) *The Natural History of Chronic Bronchitis and Emphysema*. Oxford University Press, Oxford.

4. ALTOUNYAN R.E.C. (1964) Variation of drug action on airway obstruction in man. *Thorax* **19**, 406.

5. GRANT R. (1970) The physiological basis for increased exercise ability in patients with emphysema, after breathing and exercise training (a review of the literature). *Physiotherapy* **56** (12), 541.

6. HOOPER A.E.T. (1967) Physical therapy for an emphysematous patient. *Proceedings of the 5th WCPT International Congress*, 119.

7. MCGAVIN C.R., GUPTA S.P. & MCHARDY G.J.R. (1976) Twelve-minute walking test for assessing disability in chronic bronchitis. *British Medical Journal* i, 822.

8. MUNGALL I.P.F. & HAINSWORTH R. (1979) Assessment of respiratory function in patients with chronic obstructive airways disease. *Thorax* **34**, 254.

9. MCGAVIN C.R., GUPTA S.P., LLOYD E.L. & MCHARDY G.J.R. (1977) Physical rehabilitation for the chronic bronchitic: results of a controlled trial of exercises in the home. *Thorax* **32**, 307.

10. MCGAVIN C.R., MCHARDY G.J.R. & LLOYD E.L. (1976) *Exercise can help your breathlessness*. Chest, Heart and Stroke Association, London.

11. MCGAVIN C.R., NAOE H. & MCHARDY G.J.R. (1976) Does inhalation of salbutamol enable patients with airway obstruction to walk further? *Clinical Science and Molecular Medicine* **51**, 12p.

12. WEBBER B.A., SHENFIELD G.M. & PATERSON J.W. (1974) A comparison of three different techniques for giving nebulised albuterol to asthmatic patients. *American Review of Respiratory Disease* **109**, 293.

13. LOPEZ-VIDRIERO M.T., COSTELLO J., CLARK T.J.H., DAS I., KEAL E.E. & REID L. (1975) Effect of atropine on sputum production. *Thorax* **30**, 543.

14. PIERCE R.J., ALLEN C.J. & CAMPBELL A.H. (1979) A comparative study of atropine methonitrate, salbutamol, and their combination in airways obstruction. *Thorax* **34**, 45.

15. CONNOLLY C.K. (1975) Method of using pressurized aerosols. *British Medical Journal* iii, 21.

16. McGAVIN C.R. (1976) A modified aerosol inhaler for teaching technique. *Lancet* ii, 1227.

17. PRYOR J.A. & WEBBER B.A. (1979) An evaluation of the forced expiration technique as an adjunct to postural drainage. *Physiotherapy* **65**, (10), 304. *Erratum:* p. 304, col. 2, line 7 '. . . combined with chest compression, performed by the patient alone'. *should read* '. . . combined with chest shaking and percussion by the physiotherapist.'

18. FITCH K.D. & MORTON A.R. (1971) Specificity of exercise in exercise-induced asthma. *British Medical Journal* iv, 577.

19. HARTLEY J.P.R. (1979) Editorial: Exercise-induced asthma. *Thorax* **34**, 571.

20. KILHAM H., TOOLEY M. & SILVERMAN M. (1979) Running, walking, and hyperventilation causing asthma in children. *Thorax* **34**, 582.

21. THOMPSON B.J. (1978) *Asthma and Your Child.* 5th new revised edition. Pegasus Press, Christchurch, New Zealand.

22. PRYOR J.A., WEBBER B.A., HODSON M.E. & BATTEN J.C. (1979) Evaluation of the forced expiration technique as an adjunct to postural drainage in treatment of cystic fibrosis. *British Medical Journal* ii, 417.

23. ROSENBLUTH M. & CHERNICK V. (1974) Influence of mist tent therapy on sputum viscosity and water content in cystic fibrosis. *Archives of Disease in Childhood* **49**, 606.

24. CHANG N., LEVISON H., CUNNINGHAM K., CROZIER D.N. & GROSETT O. (1973) An evaluation of nightly mist tent therapy for patients with cystic fibrosis. *American Review of Respiratory Disease* **107**, 672.

25. WOLFSDORF J., SWIFT D.L. & AVERY M.E. (1969) Mist therapy reconsidered; an evaluation of the respiratory deposition of labelled water aerosols produced by jet and ultrasonic nebulizers. *Pediatrics* **43**, 799.

26. WOOD R.E., WANNER A., HIRSH J. & FARRELL P.M. (1975) Tracheal mucociliary transport in patients with cystic fibrosis and its stimulation by terbutaline. *American Review of Respiratory Disease* **111**, 733.

27. MATTHEWS L.W., DOERSHUK C.F., WISE M., EDDY G., NUDELMAN H. & SPECTOR S. (1964) A therapeutic regimen for patients with cystic fibrosis. *Journal of Pediatrics* **65**, 558.

28. GIBSON G.J., EDMONDS J.P. & HUGHES G.R.V. (1977) Diaphragm function and lung involvement in systemic lupus erythematosus. *American Journal of Medicine* **63**, 926.

7 Surgical conditions

PULMONARY SURGERY

This section deals primarily with physiotherapy associated with surgery of the lungs and pleura, but also includes oesophageal and diaphragmatic surgery and correction of chest deformities. The general principles of physiotherapy are considered first and then details for the individual operations follow (p. 73).

Physiotherapy has an important part to play in the care of patients following pulmonary surgery and one of the aids to a quick recovery is adequate pre-operative training. The principles of pre-operative treatment are the same for all patients undergoing pulmonary surgery, but obviously vary in detail according to the individual's condition and the operation performed. Most patients are admitted a day or two before the operation and treatment should start as early as possible.

Before starting pre-operative treatment, the physiotherapist should examine the patient's medical history and chest radiographs and any other relevant investigations such as respiratory function tests. It is important at this stage that the physiotherapist evaluates the patient's normal breathing pattern and his thoracic mobility. These observations should be recorded, as they will be of value in the post-operative phase.

Aims of physiotherapy following pulmonary surgery

1 To preserve adequate ventilation.
2 To assist removal of excess secretions from the airways and thereby prevent post-operative pulmonary collapse.
3 To maintain or regain full expansion of the remaining lung tissue.
4 To assist the circulation of the legs and thereby help prevent post-operative venous thrombosis.
5 To maintain mobility of the shoulders, shoulder girdle, spine and chest.
6 To prevent postural defects.
7 To restore exercise tolerance.

PRE-OPERATIVE TRAINING

1 Explanation to the patient

During the pre-operative period, the physiotherapist should gain the patient's confidence in order that he will be prepared to co-operate after his operation, despite discomfort.

It must be explained that to maintain adequate ventilation of the lungs, breathing exercises must be performed which will inevitably be uncomfortable. He should be told that although sedation will be given, this does not eliminate pain entirely. He must understand the importance of clearing secretions present in the airways after surgery, in order to prevent post-operative complications. Reassurance must be given that deep breathing, huffing, coughing and moving around in bed, will in no way harm the stitches, drainage tubes or operation site.

The patient should also realise the importance of starting his exercises as soon as he recovers consciousness after surgery and that physiotherapy is of the greatest importance during the first few post-operative days.

2 Removal of secretions

The lungs should be as clear as possible before surgery and any excess secretions should be removed by appropriate postural drainage. If bronchiectasis is present, intensive physiotherapy will probably be necessary.

Cigarette smoking causes bronchoconstriction and excess secretions and the patient should be encouraged to stop smoking.

Bronchitis often co-exists with bronchial carcinoma and some patients may be too dyspnoeic to tolerate the true postural drainage positions for the lung bases; in such instances a modified form should be used (p. 24).

3 Breathing exercises

(a) DIAPHRAGMATIC BREATHING (p. 13).

This exercise assists the loosening of secretions by aerating the lower zones of the lungs. Encouragement should be given to relax the upper chest and shoulder girdle in order to perform the exercise correctly.

(b) UNILATERAL LOWER THORACIC EXPANSION (p. 15).

A lateral thoracotomy is used for the majority of operations included in this section. For all such operations, with the exception of pneumonectomy, the patient will be required to emphasise lower lateral thoracic expansion for the side of the incision, since movement of this side will be inhibited by pain. Unilateral expansion of the unaffected side should also be practised. Holding full inspiration for one or two seconds, during each breath taken, helps in aeration of the alveoli.

At the present time, most pulmonary surgery is performed for bronchial carcinoma. The surgeon may not always be able to predict the extent of an operation until the chest has been opened. Lobectomy may be possible, or it may be necessary to remove the entire lung. Occasionally the growth is so extensive as to make the case inoperable. It is best to prepare the patient as for a lobectomy, but to warn him that post-operatively he may have to rest the operation side for a few days and concentrate on the other side (in case a pneumonectomy is performed). Reassurance must be given that he will be told exactly what to do when he recovers from the anaesthetic. The physiotherapist is then able to avoid answering awkward questions as to the precise nature of the operation. It is the surgeon, not the physiotherapist, who should tell the patient the details of the operation.

(c) APICAL EXPANSION (p. 16).

This exercise assists re-expansion of remaining lung tissue, helps to prevent the formation of an apical airpocket and prevents a flattening deformity of the upper chest.

In summary, pre-operatively all patients should be taught: (a) diaphragmatic breathing; (b) unilateral lower thoracic expansion for both sides of the chest, with special emphasis on the incision side (except for those *known* to be undergoing pneumonectomy); (c) apical expansion for the operation side (except for pneumonectomy).

4 Effective huffing and coughing

Huffs and coughs combined with relaxed diaphragmatic breathing help to loosen and clear bronchial secretions. Many patients find huffing more comfortable than coughing. Huffing at high lung volume can be a substitute for much coughing, whereas huffing from mid lung volume to low lung volume is used to clear progressively deeper portions of the airways.

The patient must be aware of the difference between an effective huff or cough and a noise created in the throat. The physiotherapist should attune herself to the various sounds that patients make, so that she is not misled by a dry coughing noise when secretions might be heard and shifted if the huff or cough was deeper and more effective.

The physiotherapist should show the patient how she will support the chest firmly just below the incision for a lateral thoracotomy (fig. 60), and how he can support himself in order to relieve the discomfort when huffing and coughing after the operation. He should place the arm of the unaffected side across the front of the chest, the hand giving pressure just below

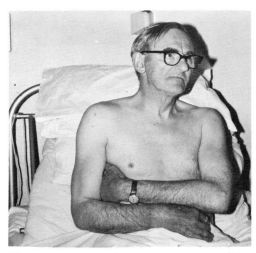

Fig. 61. *Lateral thoracotomy supported by patient.*

the incision and the other elbow giving pressure inwards to the chest wall (fig. 61).

A series of appropriate breathing exercises (in groups of four to six with a slight pause after each breath to prevent hyperventilation) should be practised by the patient three or four times a day during the pre-operative period. These should be followed by one or two effective huffs and coughs.

5 Foot and leg exercises

All patients should be taught simple foot exercises and knee flexion and extension in order to assist the circulation and help prevent post-operative venous thrombosis. The importance of practising these movements several times during every waking hour until he is able to walk around in the ward, should be stressed to the patient.

6 Posture

The habitual standing posture of the patient should be noted in order that a comparison

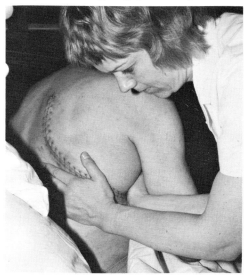

Fig. 60. *Lateral thoracotomy supported by physiotherapist.*

66

can be made with posture during the post-operative period.

Patients are ambulant very soon after surgery and problems of postural deformity rarely arise, but children and young adults sometimes find difficulty in maintaining good posture after lateral thoracotomy. The tendency to side-flex the trunk towards the incision and to lower the affected shoulder should be pointed out to the patient. The importance of correcting this tendency and thereby preventing any permanent defect, should be explained (fig. 62).

7 Arm and shoulder girdle movements

Any restriction in shoulder joint movement should be recorded pre-operatively. The prevention of loss of joint range and mobility by early post-operative shoulder girdle and arm exercises should be explained to the patient. Simple shoulder girdle and arm exercises should be practised briefly. Resisted movement with proprioceptive neuro-muscular facilitation techniques are helpful in gaining full range with minimal pain; it is of value to practise a few movements with this technique pre-operatively.

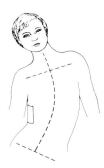

Fig. 62. *Postural defects after thoracotomy.*

8 Moving in bed

It is helpful to show the patient how to move himself up the bed taking his weight on his unaffected arm so that he can be mobile without pulling on his drainage tubes and causing pain.

POST-OPERATIVE TREATMENT

Before starting treatment, the physiotherapist should read the operation notes to find out the details of the procedure performed.

Before each treatment the patient should be observed and his record charts studied:
1 Colour, cyanosis.
2 Respiratory rate.
3 Temperature and pulse.
4 Blood pressure.
5 Drainage from pleural drain; bubbling or swing in bottles.
6 Blood gas results if available.
7 Sputum expectorated; colour and quantity.
8 Chest radiograph.
9 Analgesia; note the time the last dose was given.
10 It is helpful to listen to the breath sounds before and after treatment.

During the first two post-operative days the patient should be encouraged to do his breathing exercises, huffing, coughing and leg movements for a few minutes at least every hour that he is awake. He should also practise his arm movements three or four times during the day. It is beneficial if the night nurse is able to remind the patient to do his breathing exercises and to huff and cough when she has to waken him for nursing procedures.

DAY OF OPERATION

Post-operative treatment should start after return to the ward, when the patient is sufficiently conscious and co-operative. He should be encouraged to do his breathing exercises and then, while firmly supported, be helped to huff and cough. Often he will cough better at this stage than on the following day as there may be residual analgesia and sedation from the anaesthetic.

FIRST AND SECOND DAYS AFTER OPERATION

Treatment is probably necessary four times during the day. The patient should be sitting up in bed with the back well supported by pillows, so that there is no kyphosis or scoliosis to inhibit diaphragmatic and chest movement. After about twenty-four hours the patient will normally be allowed to sit out of bed in an armchair for short periods. The exercises can be carried out satisfactorily in this position.

Treatment should include:

1 Breathing exercises

(a) Diaphragmatic breathing.
(b) Unilateral lower thoracic expansion for both sides of the chest with emphasis on the operation side (except after pneumonectomy).
(c) Apical expansion if appropriate.
It is essential at this stage to obtain full re-expansion of the remaining lung tissue and to prevent retention of excessive secretions that might cause segmental or lobar collapse.

2 Huffing and coughing

Effective huffing and coughing, as taught pre-operatively (p. 65), must be encouraged with the chest firmly supported. The patient often finds it easier while sitting forwards in bed away from the pillows. When helping to sit the patient forward, support should be given behind the neck to avoid pulling on the painful arm.

If bronchospasm is present, a bronchodilator may be necessary before treatment.

3 Shoulder movements

Shoulder movements should be started the morning after the operation. Resistance given with proprioceptive neuromuscular facilitation techniques is helpful in achieving a good range of movement with minimal pain.

4 Foot and leg exercises

The exercises taught pre-operatively should be practised and the patient should be reminded to do each exercise 5–10 times every hour that he is awake.

5 Postural drainage

If the chest radiograph is satisfactory, the breath sounds adequate on auscultation, and the patient able to breathe deeply and huff and cough effectively, there is probably no need to put him through the unnecessary discomfort of postural drainage.

If the patient is having difficulty clearing bronchial secretions, postural drainage will probably be necessary. Some surgeons leave the decision to the physiotherapist, others prefer to be consulted first.

A patient suffering from bronchiectasis should have postural drainage.

The drainage position helpful at this stage (except for pneumonectomy, p. 74) is for the lateral basal segment of the affected lung base. The patient is positioned in side lying turned on to his unaffected side, supported by pillows and the foot of the bed raised. The degree to which the bed is tipped depends on the condition of the patient. The shoulder should not rest on the head pillows and the arm on the operated side should be supported by a pillow. Another pillow should be placed behind the back under the drainage tubes to give further support.

Analgesia

Analgesics are given at regular intervals during the first 48 hours after surgery in order to reduce pain without producing respiratory depression. If the patient is in pain and unable to perform the breathing exercises adequately, the physiotherapist should ascertain whether more analgesia can be given and carry out the treatment when it has taken effect.

Inhalational analgesics such as Entonox or Penthrane may assist effective breathing exercises.

Humidification

High humidity by means of inhalation before physiotherapy may help in loosening tenacious secretions (p. 108). A simple steam inhalation may be effective provided the patient inspires deeply, but precautions must be taken to avoid spilling the hot water.

The patient may be dehydrated at this early stage and sometimes a drink helps with coughing and expectoration.

Drainage tubes

After most operations with lateral thoracotomy incisions there will be at least two drainage tubes from the pleural cavity to underwater seal drainage bottles. The basal tube mainly drains fluid and the apical tube allows air leaking from lung tissue into the pleural space to escape, thereby keeping the lung expanded. The basal tube is normally removed within 24 hours of surgery. The apical drain (or drains) remains until there is no air leak; this is noted by any air bubbling through the drainage bottles during coughing. If it is removed too early, a pneumothorax results and another tube may have to be inserted.

Each tube is connected via an air-tight bung to a bottle partly filled with sterile water so that air cannot enter the pleura. This is known as an underwater seal. The bottle also has an open tube to allow displacement of air. As air comes out of the pleural cavity it bubbles through the water and out of the bottle (fig. 63).

To help keep the remaining lung expanded, the exit tube is usually connected to a suction pump so that a negative pressure is maintained in the bottle. The negative pressure should be increased if a large air leak is present.

If no suction pump is used, there is still a slight negative pressure in the pleural space which sucks the water a little way up the

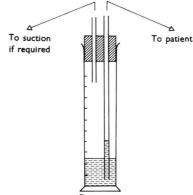

Fig. 63. *Underwater seal drainage.*

glass tube in the drainage bottle. The fluid level should swing freely with the patient's breathing.

The drainage tubes from the patient to the bottles should be long enough to allow free movement both in bed and out of bed into a chair. The patient should be encouraged to move about as much as possible. The tubes should not be clamped during physiotherapy; care must be taken not to pull and disconnect them during movement or to allow them to become kinked.

The tubes should be clamped if it is necessary to move the drainage bottles above the level of the patient, for example during transit or when transferring the bottles to the other side of the bed. If a large air leak is present, the clamp should be released as quickly as possible.

If by accident a tube should become disconnected, the part connected to the patient should be clamped and reconnected to the drainage bottle immediately. The clamp should then be removed and the fluid level checked. If there is any cause for concern the medical staff should be informed.

If a patient has a persistent apical air pocket, and the drainage tube is still in place, it may be helpful to give him breathing exercises (apical expansion) lying on his unaffected side with the foot of the bed elevated to about 45 cm (18 in).

N.B. This system of drainage tubes does not apply to penumonectomy cases (p. 75).

Intermittent Positive Pressure Breathing (IPPB)

If the patient retains secretions and is unable to cough effectively despite all methods described above, it may be necessary to combine treatment with IPPB to assist lung expansion and mobilisation of secretions (p. 95). Pressure must be kept low (below 14 cm H_2O) to prevent an increase in air leak and the treatment must only be given with the agreement of the surgeon concerned.

Naso–pharyngeal suction

If a patient is still unable to cough effectively and has sputum retention, naso-pharyngeal suction will be required to stimulate coughing and assist in removal of secretions (p. 94).

It must be emphasised that this is very rarely necessary and is unpleasant for the patient.

THIRD DAY AFTER OPERATION

The number of treatments are reduced according to the patient's condition; 3 or even 2 treatments will probably be sufficient but the patient must continue to practise his exercises several times a day.

Treatment includes:

1 Breathing exercises as above. These can be carried out sitting in a chair. As soon as unilateral expansion of the affected side is achieved, bilateral expansion (p. 16) can be added (pneumonectomy excepted).

2 Effective huffing and coughing.

3 Postural drainage if necessary. Moderately vigorous activity, e.g. climbing stairs or walking immediately prior to postural drainage is helpful in loosening secretions by stimulating deeper breathing. Drainage is discontinued when the radiograph shows satisfactory re-expansion and sputum has decreased.

4 Shoulder girdle and shoulder movements. Exercises should include active movements through as full a range as possible. When the drainage tubes have been removed, full range of motion should be achieved.

5 Foot and leg exercises are continued until the patient is walking around several times a day.

6 Posture is corrected if necessary.

7 Simple trunk mobility exercises can be included.

8 Walking and increasing activity should be encouraged.

FOURTH DAY ONWARDS

Exercises as for the third day should be continued, but the number of sessions with the physiotherapist should be reduced as soon as possible. Walking upstairs should be introduced when the patient is fit enough. Controlled diaphragmatic breathing with walking should be taught when necessary.

BEFORE DISCHARGE

Thoracic expansion (except following pneumonectomy), shoulder mobility and posture should have returned to normal. Exercise tolerance should be restored and after operations such as decortication of the lung and plication of bullae it may be markedly improved.

The patient should continue breathing exercises for 3–4 weeks following the operation, although he will probably be discharged after 10–14 days. These should consist of thoracic expansion exercises to the appropriate areas to help in restoring maximum respiratory function and to prevent chest deformity.

COMPLICATIONS OF PULMONARY SURGERY

1 Sputum retention

This is the most common complication of pulmonary surgery. If secretions are not removed, collapse of varying sized areas of lung tissue may follow. Physiotherapy is aimed at preventing this complication, but if it should occur intensive physiotherapy is essential (see previous section).

2 Persistent pneumothorax

If an air leak persists for more than forty-eight hours following surgery, an alveolar or bronchiolar leak should be suspected. The leak occurs from alveoli or bronchioli adjacent to the area of lung resected. A pneumothorax may be visible radiologically. Alveolar leaks heal quickly once the raw surface of lung comes against the chest wall, but bronchiolar leaks persist longer and may require resuturing.

It may be necessary to insert another tube if the drainage tube has already been removed and air is accumulating in the pleural cavity. If no drainage tube is in place and the pneumothorax is increasing in size, a tension pneumothorax may develop, and physiotherapy should be discontinued until an intercostal tube has been reinserted.

If a pneumothorax is allowed to remain for a prolonged period, it is a potential source of infection and may result in an empyema. If a small apical pneumothorax is present (with or without a drainage tube in place), expansion exercises should be given, particularly over the apical area and the patient should be instructed to hold full inspiration slightly longer than usual. In the case of a large apical pneumothorax (with a drainage tube in place) showing no signs of reduction in size, the patient should be positioned on his unaffected side with the foot of the bed raised to a height of about 50 cm (20 in). In this position, expansion exercises for the apical area should be practised; this may assist in reducing the air space.

3 Surgical emphysema

If air pressure builds up in the pleural space as a result of a communication between the lungs and pleura, air may track into the tissue layers producing subcutaneous or surgical emphysema. A crackling sensation is apparent when the area is palpated. It usually starts around the site of a drainage tube or suture line and may spread into adjacent tissues causing swelling of the chest wall and neck, extending in severe cases to the face and eyelids.

This condition usually subsides with correct tube management, but the physiotherapist must take care not to aggravate the condition. During coughing the glottis is closed and the intrathoracic pressure raised; therefore more air is likely to escape into the tissues. Energetic coughing must be avoided if this is increasing the surgical emphysema. Loosening and removal of bronchial secretions that are present must be assisted by breathing exercises and huffing, without coughing.

4 Bronchopleural fistula

A bronchopleural fistula is a communication between the bronchus and pleural cavity. This is a hazardous complication and usually occurs as a result of infection and disruption of the bronchial stump a week or ten days after pneumonectomy, or more rarely after lobectomy.

The signs of a fistula are: a sharp rise in pulse rate, swinging temperature, irritating cough and increase in sputum which may be blood stained. This may be followed by the sudden expectoration of large amounts of brown foul smelling fluid and eventually pus from the infected space.

Treatment consists of aspiration of infected fluid or the insertion of a drainage tube, instillation of antibiotics and postural drainage. Care must be taken to avoid infecting the remaining lung tissue. Resuturing of the bronchial stump may be necessary if healing does not occur. With bronchopleural fistula after pneumonectomy there is a serious risk of flooding the remaining lung with infected pleural fluid. It is essential that the physiotherapist keeps the remaining lung clear and great care must be taken when positioning the patient to prevent any 'spill over' of fluid. The patient should always turn with the affected side at a lower level than the unaffected side.

Following lobectomy, both sides should be drained with the patient in the prone position in order to prevent any 'spill over'. Once the fluid has been drained by insertion of an intercostal tube, it may be safe to drain the remaining segments of the affected lung in the orthodox postural drainage positions. The affected side should be drained first and the unaffected side drained afterwards in case there has been any 'spill over'.

5 Pleural effusion

A certain amount of blood stained effusion always collects after resection and the purpose of the basal tube is to drain this fluid. Aspiration may be necessary if fluid reaccumulates after removal of the drainage tube. If excess fluid is allowed to remain, fibrin will be deposited on the visceral pleura causing thickening and restriction of movement. Expansion exercises should be given to the affected area.

6 Haemothorax

In rare cases, haemorrhage into the pleural cavity may occur. This is known as haemothorax. Re-operation may be necessary to seal off bleeding points and remove blood clot from the pleural cavity. Once bleeding has been controlled, breathing exercises should be given to avoid restriction of chest movement due to pleural thickening.

INDIVIDUAL SURGICAL CONDITIONS

Lobectomy

Resection of one or more lobes of a lung.

The pre- and post-operative treatment is as already described.

If the lobectomy is for bronchiectasis, postural drainage is an essential part of the treatment both before and after surgery.

After lobectomy there will be some displacement of the bronchi as the remaining lung expands to fill the space. One must therefore adjust postural drainage positions to find the optimal position for each individual patient.

A simple lobectomy may be performed for bronchial carcinoma, but if the neoplasm has spread into the main bronchus the surgeon may perform a *lobectomy by 'sleeve resection'*. This technique has been devised in order to clear as much tissue as possible into which the neoplasm may have spread, whilst preserving maximum lung function. An end-to-end anastomosis of the main bronchus with the lower lobe bronchus is performed after resecting the affected portion (fig. 64). The patient is more likely to have difficulty in clearing sputum after this type of operation as the anastomosis may be oedematous and partially occlude the airway. There may be some bleeding into the lower lobe causing thick blood stained secretions. The principles and means of treatment are the same as far a simple lobectomy.

If a bronchial neoplasm has invaded the chest wall, it may be necessary for the surgeon to perform a *lobectomy with partial resection of the chest wall*. In these cases paradoxical chest movement may occur. This is an indrawing of the resected area of chest wall during inspiration with ballooning of the area on expiration. Breathing exercises become difficult and ineffective in these circumstances and a firm 'paradox pad' should be applied to the area to correct this movement. The pad should be made of cotton wool or similar material and be strapped firmly into position.

Severe pain is experienced when a section of the chest wall is resected and analgesia before physiotherapy is of particular importance.

Segmental resection

Removal of a segment of the lung.

A segmental resection may be performed to remove diseased areas of tuberculous lung tissue, non-malignant tumours or cysts.

The pre- and post-operative physiotherapy is in the general description (p. 64). Although only a small area of lung tissue is removed, the adjoining lung may be affected by surgical trauma during the operation causing

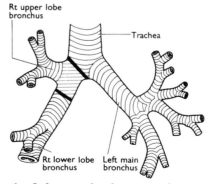

Fig. 64. *Lobectomy by sleeve resection.*

73

more secretions to form. There may be a larger air leak and more exudate draining from the pleural cavity after this operation than after a simple lobectomy. It is common to have blood stained sputum for at least a week after surgery.

Wedge resection

A very small area of lung is removed in order to resect small, non-malignant tumours or cysts such as hamartoma or small hydatid cysts. There is usually no problem with air leak or excessive exudate, but patients are likely to have a moderate amount of sputum.

Pneumonectomy

Total excision of one lung.

The extent of operation required for bronchial carcinoma is uncertain until the thorax has been opened and this has been discussed (p. 65). There are other conditions such as tuberculosis or bronchiectasis for which a pneumonectomy may be necessary. If a patient is definitely scheduled for a pneumonectomy, the physiotherapist can be more precise in pre-operative instructions.

PRE-OPERATIVE TRAINING

This should include:
1   Explanation of aims of physiotherapy.
2   Removal of secretions if present.
3   Breathing exercises.
    (a) Diaphragmatic breathing.
    (b) Lower thoracic expansion for the unaffected side.
4   Huffing to loosen secretions.
5   Effective coughing.
6   Foot and leg exercises.
7   Posture.
8   Arm and shoulder girdle movements.

POST-OPERATIVE TREATMENT

The treatment is essentially the same as that described previously (p. 67). The following points should be noted:
1   Some patients find difficulty in coughing and tend to strain. It is important to avoid straining during coughing owing to the risk of breakdown of the bronchial suture line and resultant bronchopleural fistula. Patients should therefore loosen the secretions by correct breathing exercises and huffing.
2   If postural drainage is necessary, the patient should lie as far over on to the operated side as possible, supported by pillows and with the foot of the bed raised.

A large defect in the pericardial wall may have been left and under some circumstances the heart can herniate through this defect into the pleural cavity. This distortion of the heart and great vessels can cause shock. The institution of postural drainage following a radical pneumonectomy should therefore be discussed with the surgeon concerned.
3   The patient should not lie on the unaffected side for at least ten days after the operation, i.e. until fibrin has formed in the pneumonectomy space and the danger of bronchopleural fistula has passed.
4   Bilateral lower thoracic expansion exercises may be started at the end of the first week to prevent future flattening and rigidity of the chest wall. Equal movement should obviously not be expected.
5   The patient normally sits in a chair within twenty-four hours of the operation and walks within two or three days. If the post-operative progress is satisfactory, walking up stairs can be started within one week, but this depends on the condition of each individual patient. Controlled breathing with walking, on the level and up stairs, should be taught if the patient is dyspnoeic on exertion.

Some surgeons leave a drainage tube in the pleural cavity connected to an underwater seal, for approximately twenty-four hours. This tube remains clamped and is only released for approximately one minute every hour according to instructions. Suction is never applied.

The function of this tube is to control the amount of fluid remaining in the pneumonectomy space and thereby prevent mediastinal shift. If there is too much fluid in the space, there is a shift of the mediastinum towards the remaining lung causing pressure on and partial collapse of the lung. The patient becomes breathless and may develop cardiac arrhythmias due to disturbance of the heart and great vessels in the mediastinum.

If there is too little fluid in the space, the mediastinum shifts away from the remaining lung and again arrhythmias may occur. There will also be over-inflation of the remaining lung.

Deviation of the trachea indicates mediastinal shift which can be confirmed radiographically. In order to correct this, it may be necessary for the surgeon to aspirate the hemithorax and adjust the pressures with a Maxwell Box. By this means air can either be withdrawn or instilled.

Some surgeons like to adjust the fluid level in the hemithorax by routine aspiration so that it is below the level of the bronchial stump, until the danger of bronchopleural fistula has passed.

COMPLICATIONS
FOLLOWING PNEUMONECTOMY

1   *Injury to recurrent laryngeal nerve*
During radical penumonectomy, the left recurrent laryngeal nerve is sometimes damaged, or may even have to be resected. This results in inability to close the vocal cords and therefore partial loss of effective coughing power. The patient may be able to clear his secretions adequately by breathing exercises and huffing, but the addition of IPPB is often helpful, if the surgeon gives permission. Pressure must be kept low, i.e. no higher than 10 cm H_2O.

2   *Phrenic nerve paralysis*
If a tumour involves the phrenic nerve, it may be necessary to resect it causing paralysis of the diaphragm on the affected side. The patient will have an ineffective cough due to the paradoxical movement of the diaphragm. IPPB is helpful in these cases to aerate the lung more effectively and mobilise secretions.

3   *Bronchopleural fistula* (p. 72)

Thoracotomy for inoperable bronchial carcinoma

The surgeon may find on opening the thorax that the neoplasm has invaded vital organs, or is so extensive as to make lobectomy or pneumonectomy impossible. In this case the thorax is closed leaving one tube in the pleural space to drain the post-operative exudate.

Post-operative physiotherapy is the same as for lobectomy. The clearance of secretions may be made difficult if the tumour causes distortion and obstruction of the airways. The physiotherapist should bear in mind the general condition of the patient and should make every effort to clear the bronchial secretions without causing the patient undue distress. A few patients with inoperable carcinoma deteriorate rapidly and undue pressure should not be brought to bear on the patient if physiotherapy does not relieve his symptoms.

Insertion of radioactive gold grains

When a tumour has been found to be inoperable by resection, the surgeon may implant radioactive gold grains to reduce the size of the growth. This treatment is used in certain cases as an alternative to radiotherapy. It may be done either through a thoracotomy or via a bronchoscope.

With a thoracotomy the pre- and post-operative physiotherapy is the same as that for lobectomy.

Post-operatively there is a limit to the time the physiotherapist may stay in the patient's room due to the radio-activity. She must carefully divide her time to allow a few short treatments in the day, or ideally share the treatments with another physiotherapist. The maximum time allowed will increase each day. A monitoring badge should be worn.

The chest radiographs may show gross shadowing due to the radio-activity. Two or three days after surgery, sputum may increase and contain necrotic material.

If gold grains are introduced via a bronchoscope, coughing should not be forced for the first 48 hours.

Plication of emphysematous bullae

If large emphysematous bullae are occupying space in the thoracic cavity, the surgeon may perform a thoracotomy to tie off these bullae so that the normal lung tissue can expand into the area previously occupied by the cysts. Lung function will be improved as a result.

Instruction in diaphragmatic breathing with relaxation and control of the upper chest is important. The patients undergoing this type of surgery usually have severe respiratory disability and may experience distress and difficulty in expectoration during the first few post-operative days. They will probably require intensive physiotherapy. Apical breathing is unnecessary as the emphysematous patient will already be over-inflating the upper chest. Walking with controlled breathing on the level and going upstairs should be taught.

Pleurectomy

A pleurectomy may be performed if a patient suffers from recurrent pneumo-thoraces. A small thoracotomy incision is made and the parietal pleura is stripped off the lateral chest wall. As the lung re-expands, adhesions form between the chest wall and visceral pleura, preventing recurrence of pneumothorax. Blebs or bullae may be oversewn at the same time.

The basic treatment previously described is suitable, emphasising expansion exercises for the affected side. If a drainage tube is in place pre-operatively to deal with the spontaneous pneumothorax, huffing and coughing can be taught in the usual way. If there is a partial pneumothorax and no tube in place, huffing and coughing should be demonstrated only. Vigorous coughing might cause an increase in the size of the pneumothorax.

There are unlikely to be excess secretions post-operatively when the operation has been performed for idiopathic spontaneous pneu-mothorax, as there is usually no underlying lung disease. Emphasis must be on thoracic expansion exercises.

If the operation has been performed on a patient suffering from cystic fibrosis where spontaneous pneumothorax can be a com-plication, there will be a problem with tenacious secretions. Postural drainage must be started as soon as the patient regains consciousness and will be necessary at least four times a day. Extra humidity may assist expectoration (p. 106).

Abrasion pleurodesis

Abrasion pleurodesis is an alternative surgical procedure for spontaneous pneumothorax. It is performed through a small lateral thoracotomy incision, or sometimes for cosmetic reasons a small vertical mid-axillary incision is used. The pleural surface is rubbed with an abrasive material to produce an inflammatory reaction and subsequent adhesions.

Post-operatively there are one or two drainage tubes in place. Physiotherapy is similar to that for pleurectomy.

Decortication of the lung

If the pleura has become thickened and fibrosed following empyema (tuberculous or non-tuberculous) or haemothorax, the surgeon may perform a thoracotomy and strip off the thickened layers of pleura. If simpler measures have failed to eliminate an empyema cavity, this operation may consist of complete pleurectomy with excision of the empyema cavity. The lung is then free to fill the space formerly occupied by the empyema.

The basic physiotherapy for any thoracotomy applies. Pre-operatively, movement of the chest over the affected area may be very limited and there may be dramatic improvement after decortication. Rapid expansion of the lung is essential and this is achieved by applying strong suction to the drainage tubes and vigorous breathing exercises. Lower thoracic and apical expansion exercises must be emphasised and belt

exercises may be necessary to encourage expansion in the later stages of treatment (p. 16).

In patients with extensive tuberculous scarring, the lung may fail to fill the hemithorax completely at the end of the operation. The surgeon may at a later date have to consider thoracoplasty to obliterate the air space.

Lung biopsy

A biopsy of lung tissue is sometimes taken for diagnostic purposes. When it is performed by a percutaneous needle method or by the trans-bronchial method through a fibreoptic bronchoscope, physiotherapy should not be given immediately after the biopsy. Where open lung biopsy is done through a thoracotomy, physiotherapy appropriate to the post-operative management of a thoracotomy is indicated.

Thoracoplasty

This operation is now rarely required because of advances in the treatment of tuberculosis. It was used formerly as a means of producing permanent collapse of diseased lung tissue so that healing could take place. It may be used occasionally to obliterate a space in the thoracic cavity; for example in chronic empyema or following resection of lung tissue.

During surgery several ribs are resected subperiosteally. For extensive thoracoplasty, up to 8 ribs, including the first, were resected; this was carried out in two stages. When the operation is performed to obliterate a space, the first rib is not usually removed and the neck remains more stable because the scalene muscles retain their insertion.

An unsightly scoliosis will occur if correct physiotherapy is not given. It is vital that that the patient is aware of the deformity likely to occur, and be able to correct it.

PRE-OPERATIVE TRAINING

1 *Breathing exercises*

Diaphragmatic breathing, unilateral lower thoracic expansion for the affected side and effective huffing and coughing should be taught. The patient should be shown how to support the apical area of his chest when he huffs or coughs.

2 *Postural correction in front of a mirror*

The patient will tend to develop a scoliosis with the concavity in the cervical spine and the convexity in the thoracic spine on the side of the operation (fig. 65). He must be taught how to correct these tendencies by means of lateral movement of the neck towards the side of the thoracoplasty, depression of the shoulder girdle on the operation side and correct alignment of the shoulders and pelvis.

3 Retraction of the scapulae should be taught and full-range arm movements on the side of the thoracoplasty.

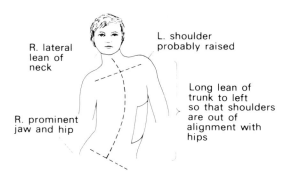

R. lateral lean of neck

L. shoulder probably raised

R. prominent jaw and hip

Long lean of trunk to left so that shoulders are out of alignment with hips

Fig. 65. *Postural defects likely after a left thoracoplasty.*

POST-OPERATIVE TREATMENT

Day of operation

Treatment is started as soon as the patient has recovered consciousness and consists of assisted huffing and coughing with firm support over the apical region of the chest wall, diaphragmatic breathing and lower thoracic expansion on the operation side. If there is paradoxical movement of the chest wall, a firm pad should be applied below the clavicle extending down into the axilla. The pad should be re-applied regularly by firm bandaging until the paradox has disappeared. Adequate analgesia must be given before physiotherapy.

1st Day

1 The pillows should be arranged comfortably.
2 Posture should be corrected, but without a mirror at this stage as it may be demoralising for the patient.
3 Diaphragmatic breathing.
4 Lower thoracic expansion on the affected side.
5 Assisted huffing and coughing with firm support, particularly below the clavicle to prevent paradox.
6 Active assisted arm movements; these are often more easily performed with a flexed elbow against resistance.
7 Depression of the shoulder girdle on the thoracoplasty side.
8 Neck lateral lean towards the thoracoplasty side; it may be helpful to give resistance below the mastoid process.

2nd Day

1 As above, but if the patient is looking better a mirror may be used.
2 Increased resistance can be used for arm movements.

3 Retraction of the scapulae.

4 Additional neck movements are included: side-flexion towards the operation side only, forward flexion and rotation.

The exercises are gradually progressed with the patient performing them sitting upright, then standing. Trunk forward flexion and side-flexion may be started after about 1 week.

Breathing exercises may be discontinued after about 1 week if there are no pulmonary complications, but postural exercises are progressed and continued until the patient is discharged from hospital. Many patients are able to maintain a good posture when standing still, but not when walking and their attention must be drawn to this. When discharged from hospital, the patient is advised to continue his exercises and posture correction, for 3 months after the date of his operation. If practical, the patient should attend occasionally for assessment and correction of posture.

TWO STAGE THORACOPLASTY

If the operation is performed in two stages, treatment is progressed as for the first stage, but the patients often have more difficulty in moving the arm. On very rare occasions the scapula is tucked in behind the 8th rib and arm elevation should be delayed until after the third day.

Surgery for diaphragmatic hernia, achalasia of the cardia (Heller's operation), oesophagectomy, ruptured oesophagus

The same principles of physiotherapy before and after surgery apply to these conditions.

A lateral thoracotomy through the sixth or seventh intercostal space is used and these lower incisions are usually more painful than the higher ones. Diaphragmatic breathing and unilateral lower thoracic expansion must be emphasised.

After surgery for diaphragmatic hernia, coughing should not be forced during the first few days.

Patients undergoing surgery of the oesophagus should not lie flat unless absolutely essential, as this may cause regurgitation of the gastric juices.

Correction of pectus excavatum and pectus carinatum

Pectus excavatum or funnel chest and pectus carinatum or pigeon chest are deformities of bone and cartilage of the thorax believed to be caused by abnormal contraction of the diaphragm.[1]

With pectus excavatum there is marked depression of the sternum, the xiphoid region being dragged inwards on inspiration. It is thought that the anterior component of the diaphragm is deficient in muscle fibres and that as the lateral and posterior fibres contract and the central tendon descends, the lower part of the sternum is pulled inwards. Many people with a mild degree of the deformity are symptom free, but it may be corrected surgically if it is causing cardio-respiratory or cosmetic problems. Various surgical techniques are used to hold the sternum forward after excision of the deformed cartilage and rib.

Pectus carinatum is a deformity where the sternum projects forward as a result of an abnormal attachment of the anterior fibres of the diaphragm. Surgical correction consists of subperichondrial excision of the prominent costal cartilages, detachment of the xiphoid and its re-attachment at a higher level on the sternum. A sub-mammary incision is usually used for these surgical procedures.

Pre-operatively unilateral lower thoracic expansion exercises for both sides of the chest are practised. Post-operatively the patient usually lies flat for at least twenty-four hours. He should not be nursed in a semi-recumbent position but should either lie flat or sit in an upright chair. Breathing exercises must be practised immediately post-operatively. The commencement of arm and trunk movements and ambulation must be discussed with the surgeon. Shoulder girdle exercises and posture correction will be necessary as soon as permission is given.

Thymectomy

Thymectomy is performed for removal of thymoma often associated with myasthenia gravis. The incision is usually a high median sternotomy.

The basic principles of pre- and post-operative physiotherapy apply, but patients with myasthenia gravis become easily fatigued and the physiotherapist should take care not to tire them. If possible, treatment should be given soon after the administration of neostigmine (or another of the anticholinesterase group of drugs).

Some myasthenic patients require ventilation post-operatively and often suffer from excess secretions which occur as a side-effect of neostigmine. Prolonged treatment cannot be tolerated and occasionally it may be necessary to cease treatment before the chest has been completely cleared in order to prevent fatigue (p. 88 for ventilator treatment).

CARDIAC SURGERY IN ADULTS

Most open heart operations are performed through a median sternotomy. These include: valve replacements, valve annuloplasty, open mitral or pulmonary valvotomy, closure of atrial or ventricular septal defect, total correction of Fallot's tetralogy, excision of ventricular or aortic aneurysm, coronary artery vein graft, removal of cardiac myxoma. Pulmonary embolectomy can be included as cardiopulmonary bypass is also necessary for this operation.

Sometimes a right thoracotomy incision is used for cosmetic reasons for the closure of an atrial septal defect.

For most closed heart operations a lateral thoracotomy is used. These include: mitral valvotomy, ligation of patent ductus arteriosus and excision of coarctation of the aorta.

A median sternotomy, or possibly bilateral anterior thoracotomy, is used for pericardiectomy.

The physiotherapist should know which incision the surgeon will use for each patient in order that emphasis can be given to exercises that will be most important during the post-operative period. Following prolonged anaesthesia there is a fall in functional residual capacity (FRC) and breathing exercises are of particular importance.

With cardiac patients, it is essential to adapt treatment to each individual's condition. A strict routine cannot be followed and it is vital never to exhaust a patient. Pre-operative training is as important as for patients undergoing pulmonary surgery. It should be started as early as possible.

Aims of physiotherapy following cardiac surgery

1   To preserve adequate ventilation.

2 To assist with removal of excess secretions in the airways.

3 To assist the circulation in the legs and thereby help to prevent post-operative venous thrombosis.

4 To maintain mobility of the shoulders, shoulder girdle and spine.

5 To prevent postural defects.

6 To restore exercise tolerance.

PRE-OPERATIVE TRAINING

1 Explanation to the patient

Explanation by the physiotherapist, in order to gain the patient's confidence and co-operation, should be similar to that described for pulmonary surgery (p. 64).

The importance of maintaining adequate ventilation of the lungs by breathing exercises and the clearance of excess secretions from the airways must be explained. Reassurance should be given that breathing exercises, huffing, coughing and moving around in bed will do no harm to the stitches, drainage tubes or operation site.

A member of the medical staff should tell the patient about the operation, including the position of drainage tubes, intravenous drip, nasogastric tube, urine catheter, electrocardiograph leads and the probability that he will need an endotracheal tube and the use of a ventilator for a few hours post-operatively. The patient should be warned that if he wakes up with an endotracheal tube in place, speaking will be temporarily impossible, but the staff will understand his requirements.

2 Removal of secretions

The majority of patients about to undergo cardiac surgery do not have excess bronchial secretions. There are, however, some patients with severe mitral valve disease or long-standing pulmonary hypertension who may have developed associated chronic obstructive lung disease and assistance with removal of secretions is required. In the earlier stage of cardiac disease the patient may have a persistent dry cough or expectorate frothy white sputum. This is not a problem that can be dealt with by physiotherapy.

If a patient has a cold or other respiratory tract infection, surgery should be postponed until the chest is clear.

If a chronic bronchitic is to have cardiac surgery he will need assistance to clear excess secretions from his airways. A modified form of postural drainage (p. 24), should be used. Care should be taken not to cause undue fatigue or dyspnoea.

The head-down postural drainage position should never be used for cardiac patients before or after surgery unless specifically requested by the surgeon concerned. This position causes an increase in venous return to the heart and an increase in atrial pressures.

3 Breathing exercises

(a) DIAPHRAGMATIC BREATHING (p. 13)

This exercise assists the loosening of secretions by aerating the lower areas of the lungs. In order to perform this exercise correctly, encouragement must be given to relax the upper chest and shoulder girdle. If a patient suffers from severe dyspnoea, relaxation and breathing control may be found easier in the high side-lying position.

(b) UNILATERAL LOWER THORACIC EXPANSION (p. 15)

For patients having a median sternotomy, expansion of the lower thorax will be inhibited after surgery and unilateral expansion of both sides of the chest should be practised in the half-lying position. Expansion for the side of the incision must be emphasised when a lateral thoracotomy is to be used.

Holding full inspiration for one or two seconds during each breath taken is useful in assisting aeration of the alveoli.

Pre-operatively, the patient should be encouraged to practise these exercises three or four times during the day. He should understand that for the first two or three days after the operation he should practise breathing exercises for at least a few minutes every hour that he is awake and not only when visited by the physiotherapist.

4 Effective huffing and coughing

Effective huffing and coughing are taught as for pulmonary surgery (p. 65). The physiotherapist should show the patient how she will support the chest over the incision and how he can support it himself. For a median sternotomy the patient can hold his hands

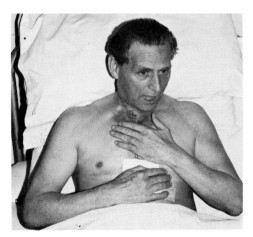

Fig. 66. *Median sternotomy supported by patient.*

directly over the front of the sternum (fig. 66) or fold his arms across the chest giving lateral support as well as pressure of the forearms anteriorly; alternatively he can hold a pillow against the anterior part of his chest. For a lateral incision the arm of the unaffected side is placed across the front of the chest, the hand giving pressure just below the incision, the other elbow giving pressure inwards to the chest wall (fig. 61).

5 Foot and leg exercises

All patients are taught simple foot exercises and knee flexion and extension in order to assist the circulation and help prevent post-operative venous thrombosis. The importance of practising these movements several times during every waking hour after surgery should be stressed.

6 Posture, shoulder girdle and arm movements

The habitual posture of the patient is noted pre-operatively and his range of arm movements. Those patients having a median sternotomy are unlikely to have difficulty with shoulder movements after surgery, but the shoulder girdle may become stiff and many patients tend to adopt a slightly kyphotic posture. Shoulder shrugging and 'shrug-circling' are useful exercises and can be practised briefly pre-operatively.

Patients having a lateral thoracotomy need arm and shoulder girdle exercises and postural correction similar to those undergoing pulmonary surgery (p. 66).

7 Pre–operative observations

During pre-operative instruction the physiotherapist should note the patient's normal chest movement, his exercise tolerance, and his habitual sleeping position. Reassurance may be necessary if the patient is required to lie flat during the post-operative period.

POST-OPERATIVE TREATMENT

Before treatment the physiotherapist must read the operation notes and the report of the patient's post-operative progress. Several observations must be made:

1 Respiration: is the patient being artificially ventilated? If not, what is the respiratory rate?
2 Level of consciousness: is the patient alert and fully responsive? Has he moved all his limbs to command since the operation?
3 Colour: is the patient cyanosed?
4 Blood pressure: has it been stable since the operation?
5 Pulse and temperature.
6 ECG: has the cardiac rhythm been stable, or have there been arrhythmias?
7 Pacemaker: is the heart being artificially paced?
8 Intra-aortic balloon pump: is this being used to assist the cardiac output?
9 Drugs: are drugs required to maintain a reasonable blood pressure? What time was the last dose of analgesic given?
10 Drains: where were the drainage tubes inserted at operation? Was the pleural cavity on either side of the chest opened?
11 Drainage: has there been excessive bleeding from any drain site?
12 Blood gas results: is the arterial oxygen tension unduly low or the carbon dioxide level unduly high?
13 Chest radiograph.
14 Auscultation: are the breath sounds satisfactory? Are there any areas of bronchial

breathing? It is helpful to listen to the chest before and after treatment.
15 Sputum: what colour sputum and what quantity has (a) been sucked from the endotracheal tube if ventilated, or (b) been expectorated by the patient?
16 Urine output: has the patient been passing urine since the operation?

Observations of this nature should be made by the physiotherapist before every treatment and any change in the general condition should be considered.

DAY OF OPERATION

If the patient is not on a ventilator, breathing exercises can be started on the day of the operation (provided the cardiovascular system is stable) as soon as he is conscious enough to co-operate. After breathing exercises, attempts at huffing and coughing should be made.

FIRST AND SECOND DAYS AFTER OPERATION

Physiotherapy will probably be necessary four times during the day. The length of treatment should be modified according to the patient's condition and should not cause undue fatigue.

1 Ventilator treatment

Many patients undergoing open heart surgery receive intermittent positive pressure ventilation via an endotracheal tube for several hours or during the first post-operative night. If there are excess secretions in the lungs physiotherapy should be given before the anaesthetist removes the endotracheal tube.

The indications for physiotherapy depend on the secretions in the lungs, the state of the circulation and the arterial oxygen tension Pa_{O_2}. Treatment with manual hyper-inflation of the lungs and gentle chest vibrations (p. 88) may be indicated, but it is probably better not employed as a routine in cardiac surgical patients. Indications for its use are the presence of well-defined areas of localised pulmonary collapse, or evidence of secretions which cannot be readily mobilised with routine suction.

Manual hyperinflation and chest vibrations can be effective in aiding removal of secretions but it may be contra-indicated since it can cause a drop in cardiac output, fall in blood pressure and sometimes a drop in Pa_{O_2}.[2] It should therefore be prescribed on an individual basis, the decision depending on the relative requirements of the circulatory and respiratory symptoms.

If the cardiovascular state is unstable, effective endotracheal suction would probable be adequate to maintain reasonably clear airways until the general condition warrants more energetic treatment.

If excess secretions are present, the physiotherapist can perform gentle vibrations in time with the normal expiratory phase of the ventilator. This may be a less efficient method of treatment, but is a suitable compromise if the cardiovascular system is not yet stable enough to justify hyperinflation.

Many patients who have undergone cardiac surgery have few bronchial secretions and need no physiotherapy at this stage.

2 Breathing exercises

If the patient is not being artificially ventilated, breathing exercises should be carried out. Those who have been ventilated should also start breathing exercises once the endotracheal tube has been removed. The patient should be sitting up in bed with the whole back supported by pillows, so that diaphragmatic and chest movements are not inhibited.

Exercises should include:
(a) Diaphragmatic breathing.
(b) Unilateral lower thoracic expansion for both sides of the chest.

If there is a median sternotomy, expansion of both sides of the chest (unilaterally) must be encouraged. If a pleural drain is *in situ*, pain may limit movement and emphasis should be given to expand that side of the chest. With a lateral thoracotomy, emphasis is given to expansion of the incision side.

If pain is severely limiting the respiratory excursion, the physiotherapist should treat the patient after an analgesic has been administered.

The patient should be reminded to practise breathing exercises at least every hour whilst awake.

3 Huffing and coughing

Effective huffing and coughing, as taught pre-operatively, must be encouraged with the chest firmly supported. The patient often finds it easier to huff and cough when sitting forward in bed away from the pillows. Great care must be taken to avoid displacing any drips or wires attached to the patient.

In the absence of heart failure or co-existent lung disease, there are likely to be fewer secretions in the airways than after lung surgery.

If the breath sounds are satisfactory, the chest radiograph reasonably clear and the patient is breathing efficiently, he will be treated in the sitting position. If there are secretions in the lungs that he is unable to clear, he should be positioned on his side and breathing exercises should be carried out, followed by huffing and coughing.

The foot of the bed should never be raised for postural drainage of a cardiac patient unless it is specifically ordered by the surgeon (p. 81).

If the patient is unable to breathe effectively, the gas exchange in the alveoli will be inefficient and there may be retention of secretions. Physiotherapy in conjunction with an intermittent positive pressure breathing machine can help to improve the gas exchange and loosen secretions (p. 95). This is often effective in the sitting position, but may be used in side-lying if necessary.

4 Foot and leg exercises

The exercises taught pre-operatively should be practised and the patient should be reminded to do these movements 5–10 times every hour that he is awake.

If an intra-aortic balloon pump is in use, bilateral foot exercises and hip and knee flexion on the unaffected side are given. Hip and knee flexion on the side of the intra-aortic balloon pump may not be given until it has been removed.

5 Shoulder movements

With a lateral thoracotomy it is important to start arm movements on the first post-operative day. With a median sternotomy these need not be started until the second day.

THIRD DAY ONWARDS

Treatment following cardiac surgery must be adapted to each individual patient's condition. The patient will start sitting out of bed from 24 hours after surgery according to his progress and the surgeon's instructions. Walking around the ward may be started as soon as the second or third post-operative day.

The number of times a day that physiotherapy is required depends on the patient's condition and it can probably be reduced to one or two treatments per day by the end of the first week.

Treatment should include:

1 Breathing exercises (as above). The patient can be positioned in side-lying if expansion is limited or breath sounds reduced. Bilateral lower thoracic expansion can be included.

2 Huffing and coughing, if secretions are present in the lungs.

3 Foot and leg exercises are given while the patient is confined to bed. These can be discontinued when he is fully mobile.

4 Arm and shoulder girdle exercises.

5 Postural correction and gentle trunk exercises if necessary.

6 Walking up stairs can usually be started about 6 days from the time of operation. This will depend on the instructions of the individual surgeon. After cardiac surgery most patients find climbing stairs much less exhausting than pre-operatively, but on occasions it is helpful to teach controlled breathing with walking on the stairs.

Treatment must be modified if any complications occur.

BEFORE DISCHARGE

Thoracic expansion, shoulder mobility and posture should have returned to normal. The patient should be increasing his exercise tolerance.

The patient should continue breathing exercises for about 3 weeks following the operation, although he will probably be discharged after 10–14 days.

COMPLICATIONS OF CARDIAC SURGERY

Following cardiac surgery, the patient will be continuously assessed by the medical staff so that any complications may be detected and appropriate treatment prescribed. Such complications include: cardiac failure, tamponade (compression of the heart by fluid or clot in the pericardium), haemorrhage, arrhythmias, and fluid and electrolyte imbalance. Other complications that particularly influence the treatment given by the physiotherapist are as follows:

1 Pulmonary oedema

Pulmonary oedema should be suspected if there is a drop in urine output, a raised central venous pressure and an increase in pulmonary secretions. Copious frothy sputum may be an early indication of pulmonary oedema. This may be white at first, becoming pink if the condition is allowed to progress.

If a patient develops acute pulmonary oedema and is being artificially ventilated, physiotherapy should be temporarily discontinued until the condition has been treated. If the patient is breathing independently, he may require assistance to expectorate the excess secretions, but medical treatment (diuretics, etc.) will be required to relieve the condition.

2 Pleural effusion

Expansion exercises must be practised in order to prevent restriction of chest movement due to thickening of the pleura. Aspiration may be needed for large effusions.

3 Breakdown of the sternal sutures

If the sternal suture line is breaking down due to infection, the patient's temperature may be raised, there may be oozing from the wound and possibly a noticeable 'click' when the patient coughs or breathes deeply. Firm support must be given to the chest during huffing and coughing, both by the staff and also by the patient when he is coughing independently. A device known as the Cough-Lok gives extra support in these instances. Care must be taken to prevent straining the suture line when the patient turns over in bed.

4 Neurological damage

Occasionally, during cardiac surgery, the brain may be damaged by embolism or anoxia. The physiotherapist must treat any form of paralysis that occurs and rehabilitate the patient as soon as possible. Obviously the patient's cardiac state may limit the form of rehabilitation.

5 Renal failure

Another rare complication of cardiac surgery is renal failure. Occasionally peritoneal dialysis will have to be instituted. Breathing exercises are particularly important to maintain function of the lung bases. Physiotherapy should be carried out during the period when the peritoneum is almost empty, in order to allow maximum basal expansion. The diaphragmatic action will be limited when the abdomen is filled with fluid and the patient will find it uncomfortable if physiotherapy is given at this time. This also applies to physiotherapy if the dialysed patient is being artificially ventilated.

PROBLEMS WITH INDIVIDUAL CARDIAC OPERATIONS

Resection of coarctation of the aorta

During the first ten days after resection of coarctation of the aorta, there are likely to be episodes of hypertension. The reason for this phenomenon is unknown, but if it occurs it could put a strain on the aortic suture line. The physiotherapist should be aware of the possibility and modify the treatment to avoid increasing the hypertension. It may be contra-indicated to lay the patient flat, even if bronchial secretions are present.

Pulmonary embolectomy

Pulmonary embolectomy may be performed for massive pulmonary embolism. Post-operative physiotherapy should be along the same lines as for any open heart operation, but pulmonary dysfunction is especially common owing to the presence of small infarcts. The patient is likely to be cyanosed and will expectorate dark brown blood stained sputum.

Manual hyperinflation with chest vibration may be indicated while the patient is artificially ventilated.

Pericardiectomy

Following this operation patients may be troubled with excessive amounts of frothy sputum and need particular encouragment with coughing. Otherwise the treatment is the same as for any closed heart operation.

Insertion of pacemaker

Pacemakers are inserted for the treatment of heart block. The incision used varies with the type of pacemaker and the preference of the surgeon concerned; it may be an abdominal incision, lateral thoracotomy, or an axillary incision. Many elderly people undergo this operation and although it is a relatively minor procedure and the pleura is not opened, the physiotherapist must give pre- and post-operative treatment to prevent any chest complications.

References

1. THOMPSON H.T. (1964) Surgical correction of sternal deformities. *New Zealand Medical Journal* **63**, 277.
2. GORMEZANO J. & BRANTHWAITE M.A. (1972) Effects of physiotherapy during intermittent positive pressure ventilation. *Anaesthesia* **27**, 258.

8 Physiotherapy for patients receiving mechanical assistance

INTERMITTENT POSITIVE PRESSURE VENTILATION (IPPV)

When a patient is being artificially ventilated via a tracheostomy or endotracheal tube (fig. 67), there are several factors, apart from the underlying disease, that predispose to excess bronchial secretions and chest infection. These include:

1 The inability to cough effectively.
2 The absence of the normal deep sigh mechanism.
3 The presence of a tube which irritates the mucous membrane.
4 The tendency for drying and crusting of

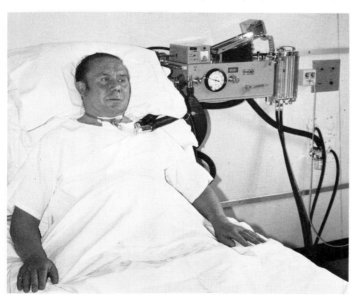

Fig. 67. *Patient being artificially ventilated via a tracheostomy tube.*

secretions and infection, due to bypass of the upper respiratory tract.

By adequate humidification and tracheal suction and care in maintaining sterile precautions, problems of excess secretions can be kept to a minimum. However, assistance with removal of secretions is often required and the most effective method is known as *manual hyperinflation with chest vibration*. It is often termed 'bag squeezing', but this name does not infer the all important type of inflation that is given.[1,2]

Manual hyperinflation with chest vibration

The patient is positioned on his side if possible and the tracheostomy tube, or endotracheal tube, is disconnected from the ventilator and connected to a manual inflation bag. One person, usually an anaesthetist, squeezes the bag, inflating the chest with a slow deep inspiration which promotes complete aeration of the alveoli. After holding the full inspiration momentarily, the bag is released quickly, to allow a high expiratory flow rate. The physiotherapist has her hands on the side of the lower rib cage and starts to compress the chest just at the end of the inspiratory period, fractionally before the bag is released. This accurate synchronisation between the two operators is essential to produce the best effect. The chest compression reinforcing the high expiratory flow rate from the bag, assists movement of the secretions in the periphery of the lung towards the main airways (fig. 68).

Approximately six deep breaths with chest vibrations are given, starting at the lung base; this is followed by suction. Suction should also precede hyperinflation if there are audible secretions in the large airways. If the patient is conscious and able to co-operate he is encouraged to attempt to cough actively when the suction catheter has been inserted, and at the same time the physiotherapist vibrates the chest to assist removal of secretions (fig. 69).

The whole procedure is probably repeated two or three times with the physiotherapist vibrating over the basal area. When that area is clear, the middle and upper areas of the chest are treated if secretions are present.

The number of times per day that treatment is performed depends both on the condition of the patient's chest and on his general condition. It may be necessary to carry it out every two hours, or even hourly, or it may only be required once or twice a day. Where possible, treatment should be timed to coincide with the nurses turning regime to avoid unnecessary discomfort to the patient.

Some form of sedation is often necessary before treatment, or treatment may be timed to coincide with sedation already prescribed.

If the secretions are thick, it is often helpful to insert 2 or 3 ml of normal saline (0·9%) into the trachea before hyperinflating the chest. The saline will go into the most dependent bronchi, and should therefore be inserted before positioning the patient to drain the affected area.

Suction of the intubated patient must be carried out with a sterile technique using either forceps or gloves. A suitable sized catheter is inserted into the endotracheal or tracheostomy tube to reach just beyond the end of the tube. Theoretically the diameter of the catheter should not be more than half

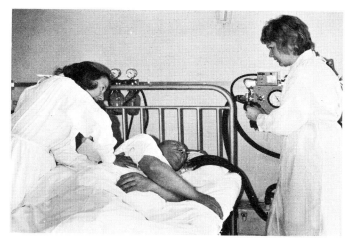

Fig. 68. *Manual hyperinflation with vibrations.*

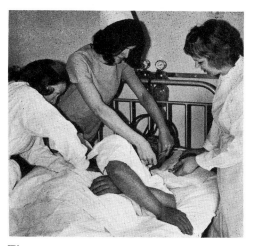

Fig. 69. *Tracheal suction with vibrations.*

the diameter of the tube through which it is passing. Either a Y-connection is used, or the catheter is pinched or left disconnected, to avoid suction until it is fully inserted. Suction is then applied and the catheter is withdrawn using a rotating action between the finger and thumb so that all available secretions are aspirated. The duration of

89

suction should not exceed fifteen seconds. The same catheter should not be used again, but is either flushed with sodium bicarbonate solution in preparation for resterilisation, or discarded if it is disposable.

If difficulty is experienced in passing the catheter down an endotracheal tube, it may be helpful to extend the patient's neck or turn his head to one side. The flexed position of the neck may cause slight kinking of the tube. It may also help to instil more saline immediately prior to suction.

Soft rubber catheters cause less trauma and are more comfortable for the patient, but may be too short for some endotracheal tubes. Where even minimal trauma would be dangerous because of a stitch line in the trachea or at the carina, it may be necessary to use Argyle Aero-flo catheters which have a specially designed tip to prevent mucosal damage.

A specimen of bronchial secretions is often required for laboratory investigations. A 'trap specimen' is collected by means of a special specimen container with a catheter attached, connected to the suction apparatus.

Equipment for inflation

There are many types of bag available for lung inflation: either the rebreathing bag attached to a ventilator may be used, or a separate hand ventilation system. It is important that the system provides a good elastic recoil when the bag is released. A 2-litre bag is normally used for adults.

Most commonly a mixture of air with a controlled quantity of added oxygen is used for hyperinflation. Provided that there is an adequate gas flow of 10–15 litres per minute, it should not be necessary to use a Waters CO_2 absorbing canister in the circuit as this can be cumbersome and heavy.[2] The analgesic effect produced by a mixture of 50% nitrous oxide and 50% oxygen (Entonox) may be helpful when carrying out this treatment.

VARIATIONS OF TREATMENT WITH SPECIFIC CONDITIONS

1 Post–cardiac surgery

The indication for treatment by manual hyperinflation with chest vibration depends on the volume of bronchial secretions present and also on the cardio-vascular state of the patient (p. 84).

If treatment is given during the first post-operative day, the patient may need to remain supine. With one hand supporting the incision, gentle vibrations are given to the side of the chest using the other hand. If the patient is treated in side-lying and has had a median sternotomy, care must be taken to avoid giving too much pressure to the lateral chest wall. The hands are placed more posteriorly than laterally and during suction the incision should be supported by one hand and forearm, while vibrating the posterior aspect of the chest wall with the other hand.

The physiotherapist must be aware of any change in the ECG pattern, or colour of the patient. The blood pressure should be taken during treatment if it has been unstable. Treatment periods should be brief as there is the danger of causing a fall in Pao_2.

2 Post–pulmonary surgery

If a patient requires IPPV following pulmonary surgery, physiotherapy with manual hyperinflation may be helpful. It can, if necessary, be combined with postural drainage for the appropriate area. It may be contra-indicated if there is a large air leak, or any sign of surgical emphysema.

3 Acute exacerbation of chronic bronchitis

There are generally copious thick secretions in the lung bases of patients with chronic bronchitis who require intubation and ventilation. Initially, vigorous physiotherapy will be needed at least every two hours. The patient can be positioned for drainage of the affected lobes before and during treatment. The chest shaking can be more energetic than with surgical patients, as there is no painful incision.

4 Asthma

Occasionally a patient suffering from asthma may be intubated and ventilated. The small airways may be plugged with bronchial casts, but manual hyperinflation and chest vibrations tend to aggravate bronchospasm and should not be started until the secretions begin to liquefy and bronchodilatation starts to occur. Some physicians order up to 10 ml of normal saline solution to be instilled before physiotherapy to assist in loosening these casts. If it is found that the treatment is aggravating bronchospasm, chest vibration on expiration should be used without manual hyperinflation, or physiotherapy may have to be withheld until there is further improvement in the patient's condition. It is often helpful to give a bronchodilator before treatment. A ventilator suitable for IPPB (p. 95) with a bronchodilator in the nebuliser can be connected to the endotracheal tube.

5 Respiratory muscle paralysis

If the respiratory muscles are paralysed, for example by acute polyneuritis or poliomyelitis, IPPV may be necessary. Manual hyperinflation is a suitable method of treatment, but 'rib springing' is often a more effective means of moving the secretions than chest vibrations in the paralysed patient.

6 Tetanus

Many patients are heavily sedated with diazepam (Valium) and artificially ventilated. Additional sedation should be given prior to physiotherapy and if there are any signs of muscle spasm, treatment should be temporarily discontinued until further sedation has been administered. Occasionally patients are therapeutically paralysed. Tetanus patients tend to have an unstable autonomic nervous system, fluctuations in blood pressure may occur and treatment may have to be adapted.

Physiotherapy includes appropriate postural drainage with manual hyperinflation and chest compression. There is often hypersecretion of mucus and areas of lobar collapse may occur. Treatments may need to be carried out every 2 hours in the early stages of the disease. Passive movements of the limbs should be given regularly and care should be taken to position them comfortably.

7 Crushed chest

If a patient with a crushed chest requires IPPV, chest shaking to the affected side is usually contra-indicated. Positioning of the patient combined with manual hyperinflation may be used with caution provided that an intercostal drain has been inserted. If there is contusion of the underlying lung there will be thick, blood stained secretions and extra saline instilled into the endotracheal or tracheostomy tube may be indicated.

Contra-indications to manual hyperinflation

Hyperinflation with chest vibrations can in some cases produce a fall in cardiac output and a lowering of the arterial oxygen tension.[3] It should only be undertaken when there is some valid indication and with the agreement of the medical staff.

The following conditions contra-indicate hyperinflation:

1 Unstable cardiovascular condition such as low cardiac output and some cardiac arrhythmias.
2 Severe hypoxaemia when few bronchial secretions are present, e.g. 'shock lung syndrome'.
3 Acute pulmonary oedema. Tracheal suction can increase pulmonary oedema, but the proximal secretions can be removed by suction as necessary. Physiotherapy should be postponed until the pulmonary oedema has been controlled by medical treatment.
4 Air leak. If there is a pneumothorax, surgical emphysema or an intercostal tube in place with a severe air leak, hyperinflation is likely to be contra-indicated. It will not be suitable for a patient with a lung condition predisposing to pneumothorax, e.g. emphysema, cystic fibrosis, irreversible fibrosis following severe 'shock lung syndrome'.
5 Severe bronchospasm. Where bronchospasm is the main problem, hyperinflation is not indicated until this has been relieved, e.g. acute asthma.

Alternative method of chest treatment

If hyperinflation is contra-indicated, but physiotherapy is required to assist removal of secretions, an alternative method may be used. The chest is vibrated in time with the expiratory phase of the ventilator instead of giving any extra inflation. The patient can be positioned, saline instilled and suction and coughing performed in exactly the same way as previously described.

Limb movements

Unconscious or paralysed patients should have passive movements to all their limbs. Active movements should be encouraged whenever possible.

For patients with neurological conditions, the basic principles for positioning, nursing and subsequent rehabilitation should be applied.

'Weaning' from a ventilator

'Weaning' from the ventilator is started when the patient's condition has improved sufficiently, and should be carried out under the supervision of the anaesthetist. The criteria usually required before a patient can be successfully weaned from a ventilator are: a clear chest radiograph, minimal non-infected sputum, normal blood gases on 40% oxygen or less, functioning gastrointestinal tract and reasonably good morale of the patient.[4] The patient may start by breathing without the ventilator for short periods and the length of time is increased according to the anaesthetist's instructions. The respiratory and pulse rates are recorded during spontaneous breathing and blood gas measurements are made intermittently. If there are signs of respiratory distress, the anaesthetist is informed and the patient is reconnected to the ventilator.

For patients breathing independently through a tracheostomy tube, humidification is essential to prevent bronchial secretions becoming thick and tenacious. An attachment to the tracheostomy tube will provide humidified air with the appropriate amount of additional oxygen.

Breathing exercises should be started during this stage to re-educate active use of the respiratory muscles. The patient should be encouraged to cough actively, instead of relying entirely on the stimulation of the suction catheter.

When the patient is breathing independently for several hours in the day, the physiotherapy would probably comprise active breathing exercises in the side-lying position with vibrations, active huffing and tracheal suction. Manual hyperinflation can be continued if necessary, but this should be stopped as soon as the patient is able to huff and cough effectively, so that he can manage without assistance once the tube has been removed.

After removal of the tube, the dressing covering the tracheostomy should be as air-tight as possible, but it is still necessary to teach the patient to hold the site of the tracheostomy firmly while coughing (fig. 70). If there is an air leak, some of the secretions

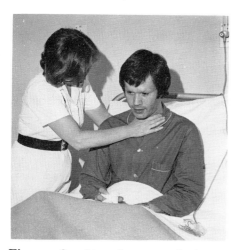

Fig. 70. *Coughing after removal of tracheostomy tube.*

and air are blown out through the incision instead of being expectorated from the mouth and the full force of the cough is wasted.

For the first forty-eight hours after removal of a tracheostomy tube, it is often necessary to increase the frequency of treatments to assist clearance of secretions. At this stage, the assistance of IPPB (Intermittent Positive Pressure Breathing) with physiotherapy may help the patient to overcome what may be a critical period (p. 101).

BRONCHIAL LAVAGE

When there is a tenacious exudate in the periphery of the lungs, either in the terminal bronchioles or alveoli, which is not responsive to the routine methods of removal (e.g. postural drainage, humidification, IPPB), the procedure known as bronchial lavage is occasionally used. The term bronchial lavage is used for two distinct procedures one involving the instillation of large volumes of solution into the bronchial tree and the other using small volumes of solution.

The procedure involving the larger volumes of fluid is indicated for the treatment of alveolar proteinosis and very occasionally may be used for intractable attacks of asthma. If the exudate in the periphery of the lungs is allowed to remain, it impairs aeration of the alveoli and inhibits gas transfer.

The aim of bronchial lavage is to flush out as much of the exudate as possible. It is a skilled procedure carried out under general anaesthesia using a double lumen tube. One lung is gradually filled to FRC (functional residual capacity) with warmed buffered

93

electrolyte solution. Further volumes of electrolyte solution are instilled and drained out aiming to keep the volume of the treated lung at FRC or approximately 500 ml above FRC. After up to 20 litres of electrolyte solution have been used, the lung is drained completely using suction and posture. The lung is then reinflated by positive pressure ventilation and a short period of post-treatment ventilatory support is often employed. Bronchopulmonary lavage is more difficult to carry out in the treatment of asthma because the solution drains out of the lungs less easily.

Following extubation, assisted breathing by use of IPPB and encouragement to cough may be necessary, and possibly postural drainage. However, when a few hours of mechanical ventilation are used after the procedure, minimal physiotherapy is required because so little fluid remains in the lungs. It has been found beneficial in the cases of alveolar proteinosis to inhale normal saline or sterile water from an ultrasonic nebuliser (p. 107) at least four times daily for a few days preceding lavage. Long-term domiciliary use of high humidity, by ultrasonic nebuliser or a heated nebuliser, has been tried for a few of these patients in an attempt to lengthen the time before recurrence of symptoms. It is possible that this may be effective.

The bronchial lavage procedure involving small volumes of solution is carried out using a fibre-optic bronchoscope. This method is sometimes employed in an attempt to remove mucous plugs in bronchopulmonary aspergillosis or asthma. Small quantities (5–10 ml at a time, up to 50–100 ml) of sterile saline are instilled down the centre channel of the bronchoscope. Viscid secretions may be liquefied and removed from the affected bronchial segments.

NASO-PHARYNGEAL SUCTION

Naso-pharyngeal suction, as a means of stimulating a cough, is an unpleasant procedure for the patient, and should only be performed when absolutely necessary. The indication for suction is the inability to cough effectively and expectorate when sputum is being retained. It may be necessary in such conditions as respiratory failure, due to acute exacerbations of chronic bronchitis (p. 44), post-operative complications, laryngeal dysfunction or various neurological disorders. Small babies not coughing effectively need naso-pharyngeal suction as part of the routine physiotherapy.

It is contra-indicated when there is severe bronchospasm or stridor.

Technique

It is better to carry out this procedure through the nose in adults, but it is sometimes easier to suction small babies through the mouth.

A soft catheter of suitable size should be lubricated with a water soluble jelly, and gently passed through the nasal passage so that it curves down into the pharynx. Effective coughing is often stimulated with the catheter in this position. Suction should not be connected until the catheter is in the pharynx.

In adults it may be possible to pass the catheter between the vocal cords and into the trachea. If the patient is able to co-operate this is easier to perform if the neck is extended and with the tongue protruding. The catheter should be inserted during the inspiratory phase and if it is passed into the trachea, vigorous coughing will be stimulated.

It is important to observe the patient for

signs of anoxia during the procedure and oxygen should be available.

If it has been difficult to insert the catheter and the patient looks cyanosed, instead of withdrawing the catheter, the suction should be disconnected and oxygen administered until the patient's colour has improved, then suction should be reconnected.

Infants should be positioned in side-lying while naso-pharyngeal suction is carried out to avoid the danger of inhalation of vomit. Adults who are nursed sitting up in bed, can be suctioned in that position, whereas comatose patients are usually suctioned while lying on their side.

Naso-pharyngeal suction is contra-indicated in patients with head injuries where there is a leak of cerebrospinal fluid into the nasal passages. Oro-pharyngeal suction through an airway is used as an alternative method.

Some authorities feel that the technique of passing the catheter into the trachea should not be used because of the risks of causing laryngeal spasm or vagal stimulation.[5] However, others find that it is a valuable technique provided that it is carried out carefully and that oxygen is always available.

Naso-pharyngeal suction is a procedure that should not be undertaken until every attempt to achieve effective coughing has failed. Alternative treatments available would be bronchoscopy, temporary intubation or tracheostomy, but these can very often be avoided by the use of careful suction.

INTERMITTENT POSITIVE PRESSURE BREATHING (IPPB)

Use of an Intermittent Positive Pressure Breathing machine (IPPB) can be extremely valuable when chest physiotherapy alone is not having the desired effect. The ventilator can provide more effective aeration of the alveoli and can promote expectoration; it is also a means of administering drugs and humidity directly into the airways. If the patient relaxes, the work of breathing is considerably reduced.[6,7] IPPB is most beneficial when it is used as an adjunct to physiotherapy; the maximum benefit is not achieved if a patient uses the machine without correct instruction.

There are several types of IPPB apparatus suitable for use with physiotherapy. At this hospital the 'Bird Mark 7' is employed, but others such as the 'Bennett TV-4' or 'PV-3P' (fig. 71) or Basic Mini-Bird (fig. 72) are also suitable. These machines are pressure-cycled ventilators driven by compressed oxygen or air. Some other models are driven electrically.

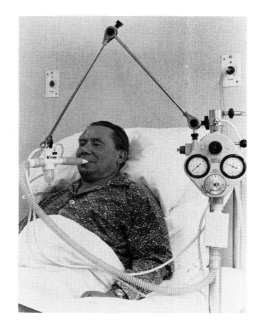

Fig. 71. *Bennett PV-3P.*

95

The essential features of an IPPB apparatus for use with physiotherapy are:

1 *Positive pressure* range of at least 0–30 cmH$_2$O.

2 *Simplicity* of controls.

3 *Portability*: the apparatus should be compact and easily movable from patient to patient.

4 *Sensitivity*: the inspiratory phase should be initiated ('triggered') by the patient with minimal effort. Fully automatic control is unpleasant for most patients and unnecessary for physiotherapy, but a hand triggering device is a useful asset on occasions.

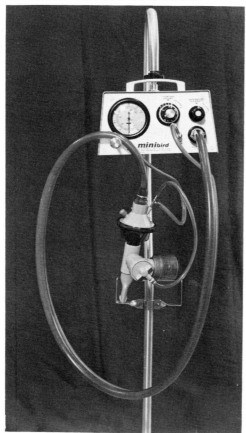

Fig. 72. *Basic Mini-Bird.*

5 *Flow control*: in machines such as the 'Bird Mark 7' the inspiratory gas is delivered at a flow rate which can be pre-set by means of a control knob. Optimal distribution of gas is achieved at relatively slow flow rates. However, if the patient is very short of breath and has a fast respiratory rate, a slow inspiratory period may be unacceptable. It will then be necessary to deliver the gas initially at a fast rate. It is important to have the facility for adjusting the flow rate to suit the individual patient.

On other machines such as the 'Bennett' there is no adjustment necessary as an automatic variable flow is provided. This is called 'flow sensitivity' and means that the flow of inspired gas adapts to the resistance of the individual patient's airways.

6 *Nebuliser*: an efficient device for nebulisation is essential. The machine must never deliver unhumidified gas. In order to provide an effective means of administering drugs the nebuliser must be capable of producing fine particles and of delivering the contents quickly (3–4 ml in 10–15 minutes). A large nebuliser (500 ml) can be fitted into the circuit if frequent and prolonged use of the ventilator is required.

7 *'Air-mix' control*: if the machine is driven by oxygen it is necessary that air is entrained in order to deliver a mixture of air and oxygen. 100% oxygen should never be delivered to the patient. Many patients with severe hypoxia require oxygen and it is dangerous to use an IPPB machine delivering air alone (p. 33). If the machine is not powered by oxygen, it can be powered by compressed air with an attachment to provide a controlled, optimal, concentration of added oxygen. With the 'Bird Mark 7', a simple method of achieving a 24% oxygen concentration is to run 2 litres of oxygen through a hypodermic needle into the inlet

port of the micronebuliser, the machine being driven by compressed air. If a non-compensated oxygen flow meter is used, the flow rate should be set at 2 litres per minute before connecting the tubing in order to obtain an accurate oxygen concentration.

The Bennett PV–3P has a diluter attachment to produce an appropriate flow of oxygen.

In the rare cases when Entonox is used to provide analgesia through an IPPB machine, the air-mix control should be in the position to provide 100% of the driving gas.

8 *Mouthpiece or mask*: the majority of patients prefer to use a mouthpiece for IPPB, but a face mask is essential for treatment of confused patients.

9 *Breathing-head assembly*: it is most economical to have several sets for each IPPB machine. A breathing-head assembly consists of a mouthpiece or mask, exhalation valve, micro-nebuliser with tubing and two channel tubing which connects the former parts to the machine.

To prevent cross infection, it is essential for each patient to have a complete breathing-head assembly which is sterilised at least every week or when the course of treatment is completed. The machine itself can be moved from patient to patient.

Preparation for treatment

1 The nebuliser is filled with the required solution. Any drug used in the nebuliser must be prescribed by the physician or surgeon in charge of the patient.

If IPPB is being used for the delivery of a bronchodilator, the prescribed dose of the drug is combined with normal saline to give a total of 3ml of solution. Normal saline solution alone may be used for humidification, but the quantity is unimportant because it is not essential to use up all the solution, or more can be added if required. Some physicians prescribe acetyl cysteine (Airbron), but in this case the machine must be driven by air as oxygen renders the substance less effective. Glycerols are unsuitable for some nebulisers.

2 The breathing-head assembly is connected to the ventilator, and the ventilator is connected to the driving gas.

3 The physiotherapist must ensure that the 'air-mix' control is in position for the entrainment of air.

4 If the machine has an 'expiratory timer' (automatic control), this is turned off.

5 The controls of the ventilator are set according to the individual's requirements. With the 'Bird Mark 7' the pressure setting is likely to be between 13 and 15 cmH$_2$O and the flow rate between 6 and 10. The aim is to adjust the pressure and flow controls to provide regular, assisted ventilation without discomfort. A patient with a rigid rib cage will require a higher pressure setting to obtain an adequate tidal gas exchange than someone with a more mobile rib cage. It is sometimes easiest to start with the pressure and flow controls set at 10 and to adjust them as the patient becomes accustomed to using the ventilator. The sensitivity control is usually adjusted to a low figure (5–7) so that minimal inspiratory effort is required. The end of the sensitivity control scale requiring greater effort is only of value when a patient with respiratory muscle weakness is being weaned from a ventilator.

With the Bennett 'PV–3P' and 'TV–4' the only control to be set is the pressure, and the nebuliser is turned on separately.

6 The ventilator is turned on to ensure that the nebuliser is functioning correctly and that there are no leaks in the breathing-head assembly.

Treatment of the patient

The position of the patient depends on the condition for which the IPPB is being given; it may be effectively used in the sitting, high side-lying, or side-lying positions (figs. 73 and 74). The patient should be comfortable and able to relax the upper chest and shoulder girdle.

The patient is told to close his lips firmly round the mouthpiece and breathe in through his mouth. After minimal inspira-

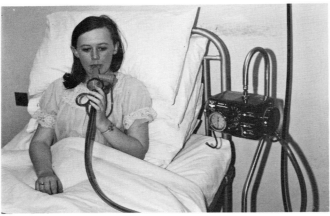

Fig. 73. *IPPB in sitting.*

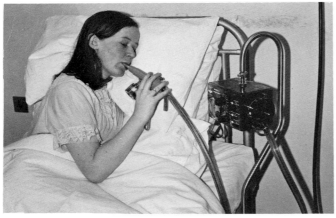

Fig. 74. *IPPB in high side-lying.*

tory effort the machine is triggered into inspiratory flow. The patient should then relax during inspiration, allowing air from the ventilator to inflate his lungs. Provided that he relaxes, the machine will cycle into expiration when the pre-set pressure is reached at the mouth. If he attempts to assist inspiration, there will be a delay in cycling into expiration; a similar delay occurs if there is any leak around the mouthpiece or mask, or from the patient's nose. It is often necessary to use a nose clip until he becomes accustomed to the ventilator.

Expiration should be quiet and relaxed; forced expiration with or without IPPB tends to increase airways obstruction (p. 14). If the patient exhales before the ventilator cycles into expiration, the needle of the pressure gauge swings round to a higher pressure than that set, while at the same time the machine cycles prematurely into expiration. The movement of the needle is a useful indicator of correct or faulty technique.

After a few breaths have been taken using the ventilator correctly, the patient is encouraged to use the lower chest during treatment. The physiotherapist places her fingers on the chest as for diaphragmatic breathing; basal expansion can also be encouraged.

IPPB, taught correctly, is not exhausting for the patient. The most common faults are the attempt by the patient to assist inspiration either by nose or mouth and premature expiration.

The exhalation valve may be provided with a retard cap which can be used to give resistance to expiration. Unless it is specifically ordered, it is preferable to remove this cap, as it can easily be placed in the wrong position and impede expiration.

To avoid hyperventilation and resultant dizziness, the patient should pause momentarily after expiration, before the next inspiration.

Treatment continues until the contents of the nebuliser are used. This takes approximately 10–15 minutes.

INDICATIONS FOR USE OF IPPB

1 Acute exacerbation of chronic bronchitis

For patients in respiratory failure due to sputum retention, which may occur during an acute exacerbation of chronic bronchitis, treatment with IPPB can be invaluable and intubation frequently avoided (p. 44).

The patient is often confused, drowsy and unable to cough effectively. With this type of patient it is often necessary to use the mask and it is helpful to have another physiotherapist or a nurse to assist with the treatment (figs. 75 and 76). If possible, the patient should be turned on to his side and the foot of the bed elevated if he will tolerate it. One physiotherapist, or the nurse, should elevate the jaw and hold the mask firmly over the patient's face ensuring an air-tight fit, whilst the other physiotherapist shakes the chest on expiration. The operator holding the mask may use the manual control on the machine in order to impose effective deep breaths on the patient. After about the first ten minutes of treatment the patient may become more rational and start to cough spontaneously, but if effective coughing is not stimulated, naso-pharyngeal suction may be necessary (p. 94).

At first, treatment should be repeated at hourly or two-hourly intervals. As the patient's condition improves, the frequency of treatment is reduced. It has been shown

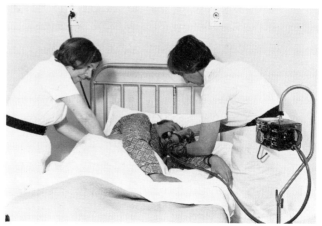

Fig. 75. *IPPB with mask.*

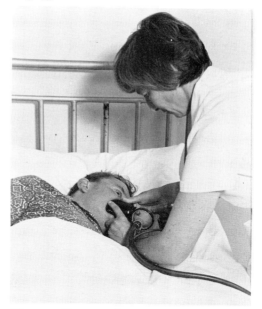

Fig. 76. *Close-up of mask.*

that a fall in arterial oxygen content can occur as a result of this treatment,[8] and therefore each session should be limited to a maximum of twenty minutes.

A bronchodilator drug is usually prescribed to be given in the nebuliser at four hourly intervals. Normal saline solution alone is used for the interim treatments.

If any increase in drowsiness is observed while treating the patient, it is probably caused by an increase in arterial carbon dioxide level due to an inadequate tidal gas exchange. The pressure and flow controls need to be adjusted to increase the tidal volume. With the Bird ventilator an increase in pressure setting will be required and probably an increase in flow rate. A drowsy patient may need encouragement to trigger the machine to maintain an adequate minute ventilation. All patients must be observed for any signs of increased drowsiness during the treatment and for a short period after treatment.

2 Relief of bronchospasm

IPPB is a useful method of administering bronchodilators, while at the same time relieving the work of breathing, as in severe acute asthma (p. 47). It is also used when a patient with bronchospasm requires mechanical assistance to loosen tenacious secretions, as in allergic bronchopulmonary aspergillosis (p. 59), or chronic bronchitis.

If bronchial secretions are present, the bronchodilator should be given in a comfortable relaxed position (high side-lying or half-lying) and physiotherapy to assist the removal of secretions should not be attempted until the bronchodilator has taken effect.

To estimate the effect of the treatment, it is helpful to record the FEV_1 and FVC, or peak expiratory flow rate, before and after treatment (p. 34).

The physician must prescribe the bronchodilator and the frequency with which it is given. Drugs commonly used are salbutamol (Ventolin) and terbutaline (Bricanyl). A dose of 5 mg (1 ml) or 2·5 mg (0·5 ml) of 0·5% salbutamol solution is used, and the dosage of 1% terbutaline is 7·5 mg or 5 mg (0·75 or 0·5 ml). Maximal response is usually achieved 15–30 minutes after inhalation.

If bronchospasm is not relieved by these drugs, 3 mg (0·3 ml of 1% solution) of atropine methonitrate may be tried. Maximal response with this drug may not be reached until 1 hour after treatment. The side-effects of these three drugs are mentioned on p. 48.

Although these dosages may appear large, it must be remembered that only between 10 and 20% of the drug reaches the patient, the rest being lost in the equipment and exhaled gas.[9]

3 Sputum retention in medical and surgical conditions

In conditions such as bronchitis or a chest infection secondary to emphysema, or in post-operative cases, the patient may breathe and cough ineffectively and retain sputum. IPPB assists the physiotherapist by giving humidity with the nebuliser and aerating the lungs more effectively, thus helping to mobilise secretions. Normal saline is used in the nebuliser unless bronchospasm is also present and the treatment can be carried out in conjunction with postural drainage. Bronchoscopy may be avoided if the secretions can be cleared. Possibly only two or three IPPB treatments will be necessary. As soon as the patient can breathe deeply enough to loosen secretions and cough effectively, physiotherapy alone is continued.

4 Following major surgery

If a patient is too ill to carry out breathing exercises efficiently, IPPB may be used to increase the tidal volume. Expansion exercises are given in conjunction to improve alveolar ventilation.

5 Laryngeal dysfunction and phrenic nerve paralysis

Occasionally the larynx is traumatised if an endotracheal tube is in place for several days. If resection of the left recurrent laryngeal nerve is necessary during radical pneumonectomy, there is difficulty in closure of the vocal cords. In both instances IPPB is found to be helpful in assisting ventilation and removal of secretions.

If the phrenic nerve has been divided during pneumonectomy (p. 75), IPPB may be necessary to assist ventilation post-operatively. The surgeon must give his permission.

6 Closure of tracheostomy

During the period of healing of a tracheostomy after 'weaning' from a ventilator, the patient may become easily fatigued and unable to clear the airways adequately. IPPB with physiotherapy may help the patient surmount this difficult period. In order for the machine to function correctly, it is often necessary to hold the tracheostomy dressing firmly to prevent any air-leak.

7 Chest deformity

Patients who have chest wall deformity and respiratory muscle weakness, such as may occur after acute poliomyelitis, are likely to have a reduced vital capacity. During chest infections, assistance will be needed to clear the airways. If the rib cage is rigid, a higher pressure setting on the IPPB machine is necessary to produce adequate ventilation.

8 Fractured ribs

Patients in road traffic accidents with fractured ribs may have underlying contused lung. If the chest wall is stable, IPPB may help mobilise tenacious blood stained secretions. The possibility of pneumothorax must be eliminated before considering this treatment. Where analgesia is ineffective a localised intercostal nerve block may relieve pain and permit effective physiotherapy.

9 Brain damage

The patient with brain damage may be unable to co-operate with the physiotherapist in maintaining clear airways. IPPB with the face mask to provide periods of effective ventilation, combined with chest vibrations, may be indicated.

10 Re-education of paralysed patients

IPPB machines with a sensitivity control can be used in the re-education of paralysed

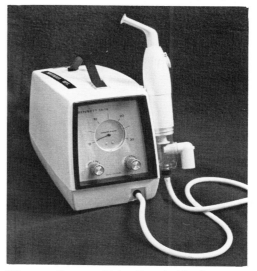

Fig. 77. *Bennett TA–1B suitable for home use.*

respiratory muscles, e.g. following acute polyneuritis. The sensitivity control is initially set at a low figure, and then gradually increased to necessitate greater inspiratory effort. In this way the machine may be used to 'wean' patients from non-triggered positive pressure ventilators.

11 Home use

A very small percentage of patients with chronic respiratory disease, who are unable to clear their bronchial secretions, require an IPPB machine at home. If it is considered that by using a machine at home, the patient will avoid admissions to hospital, it may be justified for the hospital or patient to buy one. An electrically operated ventilator such as the Bennett TA–1B (fig. 77), is usually more convenient at home unless the patient needs additional oxygen.

CONTRA-INDICATIONS TO IPPB

1 Pneumothorax

IPPB would tend to increase a pneumothorax and should therefore not be used.

2 Bullae

There is a danger of causing pneumothorax if IPPB is used for a patient with emphysematous bullae.

3 Lung abscess

There is a risk of causing air trapping in the cavity and it is inadvisable to use IPPB for this condition.

4 Haemoptysis

5 Active tuberculosis

6 Cystic fibrosis

Patients with cystic fibrosis have a tendency to pneumothoraces. IPPB should only be used at the request of the physician and the pressure should be kept low. It has also been shown to increase the residual volume in these patients after a prolonged period of treatment (p. 56).

7 Post–operative air leaks

A patient with an intercostal drain to control an air leak, who also has sputum retention, should only use IPPB with the surgeon's permission. The pressure should be kept low (no higher than 13 cm H_2O).

8 Bronchial tumour in the proximal airways

Air trapping could result if IPPB is used when a tumour is partially obstructing a large bronchus. It could be used to assist clearance of bronchial secretions if the tumour is in the peripheral airways.

9 Unnecessary use

If a patient can breathe and cough adequately without IPPB, it is a waste of time and apparatus to give treatment with IPPB.

IPPB apparatus is expensive. It is unwise to allow patients to become dependent on the machine if it is not essential. Patients should be 'weaned' from the machine as soon as it is no longer serving a genuine purpose.

Sterilisation of equipment

Each patient should have his own breathing-head assembly so that the risks of cross infection are minimised.

After each treatment the mouthpiece is scrubbed with soap and warm water and the nebuliser is rinsed and dried. The tubing is detached from the ventilator and the complete assembly stored in a polythene bag or other suitable container until required again. After the course of treatment the entire breathing-head assembly is sterilised.

To sterilise the breathing-head assembly, the mouthpiece is scrubbed and the other component parts are disassembled and rinsed; the capillary jets or tubing of the nebuliser are cleaned with the probe provided for the purpose. The separate pieces are then immersed in a suitable disinfectant for the prescribed length of time. Quats (a product of the Bird Corporation known as 'Birdbath' in the USA) or Cidex may be used. Hibitane and Phenol are not suitable for this equipment. They are then rinsed thoroughly with water to eliminate the taste of the disinfectant. A syringe should be used to flush the capillary tubing. Finally, the equipment is dried, reassembled and stored in a suitable container until required again.

If there is a shortage of equipment, the complete breathing-head assembly must be sterilised between each patient's treatment. It is not adequate to sterilise only the mouthpiece and exhalation valve.

If the breathing head assembly is sterilised in a central sterilising department the component parts should be washed and dried before packing for sterilisation.

The ventilator itself is sterilised with ethylene oxide gas.

A machine used for a patient with particularly resistant strains of bacteria, should if possible be confined to that patient. It should then be sterilised before use on any other patient.

Servicing of equipment

The IPPB machine should be cleaned internally and overhauled every three months by a specialist engineer.

It is important to keep a stock of spare parts so that any perishable or breakable parts such as rubber washers or springs can be replaced quickly.

USE OF NEBULISERS

A nebuliser is a means of administering drugs by inhalation. It breaks up the solution to be inhaled into fine droplets which are then suspended in a stream of gas. The patient can actively inhale this gas stream containing the drug instead of it being delivered by positive pressure as with IPPB.

Ideally a nebuliser should be simple, reliable, easy to clean and resterilise and inexpensive. There are several nebulisers suitable for the delivery of small volumes of solution, for example the Bard Inspiron Mini-neb, the Acorn, Turret, Hudson, Bennett twin and Bird micronebuliser.

The rate of output and particle size of the nebulised solution depends not only on the efficiency of the nebuliser, but also on the power of the driving source. If a relatively large volume is to be inhaled, or if the solution is sticky, the combination of an efficient nebuliser with a powerful driving source is important.

The nebuliser can be powered by oxygen or compressed air, the latter being obtained either from a cylinder or an electrically operated air compressor (fig. 78). Most nebulisers require a flow of 5–6 litres per minute of gas. For those patients with a raised Pa_{CO_2} who are dependent on their hypoxic drive to stimulate breathing, this concentration of oxygen may be too high and compressed air should be used.

A suitable air compressor should be oil-free, portable, durable, requiring minimal servicing and capable of producing an adequate pressure and flow of air. If sticky antibiotics are to be inhaled or quantities of drug greater than 2 or 3 ml, the pressure of one of the more powerful compressors is required (e.g. Medix Wobl Pump, Medix Minor, Medic-Aid C-50). If only a small quantity of bronchodilator is to be delivered, a compressor with lower output may be used (e.g. Medic-Aid RTU 4).

Many nebulisers are supplied fitted with a face mask. It has been shown that with a mask much of the drug is deposited on the face and in the upper respiratory tract.[10] It is therefore more efficient to use a mouthpiece, allowing an aperture in the system for entrainment of air and for exhalation. The patient is then able to keep his mouth closed round the mouthpiece throughout the inhalation treatment. It may be necessary to use a face mask for small children who are unable to manage a mouthpiece.

The patient should be in a well-supported

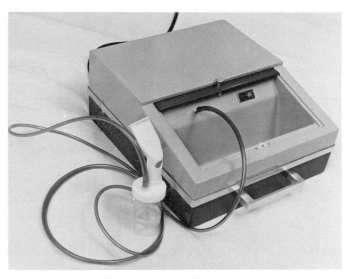

Fig. 78. *Medix Mini-Pump.*

position and with the upper chest relaxed, should attempt to do diaphragmatic breathing while inhaling from the nebuliser. A few patients tend to hyperventilate while using a nebuliser and it is helpful to suggest that two or three deeper breaths are interspersed with periods of breathing control. This technique may also provide better distribution of the nebulised particles than if using diaphragmatic breathing to a small tidal volume throughout.

INDICATIONS FOR THE USE OF NEBULISERS

1 Relief of bronchospasm

Where there is no indication for IPPB, and when the response to the drug in solution is better than with a pressurised aerosol, bronchodilator drugs are often administered by means of a nebuliser (p. 47, fig. 50).

In patients with emphysematous bullae or cystic fibrosis and other conditions where IPPB is contra-indicated, but where there is a response to bronchodilator drugs, a nebuliser is often useful.

2 Administration of antibiotics and antifungal agents

In some cases of resistant chest infections such as in cystic fibrosis, or bronchiectasis, antibiotics may be prescribed to be inhaled directly into the lungs. The nebuliser should be fitted with a one-way valve system and wide bore tubing (fig. 79) to allow the exhaled gas to be vented out through a window. This is necessary to prevent small quantities of antibiotics remaining in the atmosphere with the result that dormant organisms become resistant to the antibiotics. It is hoped that an effective filter may become available to attach to the nebuliser instead of the valve and tubing.

Antifungal drugs such as natamycin (Pimafucin), or Brilliant Green, are sometimes inhaled in the treatment of aspergilloma, or bronchopulmonary aspergillosis. In all these cases, if postural drainage is carried out, it should precede the inhalation.

3 Aid to expectoration

Some physicians prescribe mucolytic drugs, while others feel that normal saline solution, or sterile water, delivered as a mist may be equally beneficial. Normal saline is often used for patients with cystic fibrosis in conjunction with postural drainage (p. 55). It is difficult to use most small nebulisers while lying down. The Bird micronebuliser can, however, be used in any position (p. 55, fig. 59).

4 Local analgesia

Inhalation of Marcain (3–4 ml of 0·5% Marcain plain) may be useful in patients with intractable cough which may occur with fibrosing alveolitis, or viral infections affecting the irritant or cough receptors in the mucosa of the large airways. A study has shown that the period of freedom from persistent cough may last up to 6 weeks.[11] It is presumed that a reflex cycle is broken to produce this prolonged response to the drug. Treatment is repeated according to the individual's symptoms and in some cases is required as often as three times a day. It is advisable that the patient does not eat or drink for an hour and a half after the inhalation. Marcain is used in preference to Lignocaine as the analgesic effect is of longer duration and it also has a more favourable therapeutic/toxic ratio.

It has also been suggested that suppression of the J-receptors in the alveoli may relieve dyspnoea in patients with the intractable dyspnoea of severe fibrosing alveolitis, or in some terminally ill patients such as those suffering from alveolar carcinoma. Marcain has been used in an attempt to suppress the J-receptors, but no formal trial has yet been completed.

Domiciliary use of nebulisers

Patients requiring domiciliary equipment should be carefully selected and only those benefiting from treatment that cannot be given in any simpler form should be loaned equipment. Before supplying a nebuliser system for delivery of bronchodilators, accurate tests of changes in FEV_1 and FVC should be carried out to ensure that the response is significantly greater than by using a simple pressurised aerosol (p. 34). Another method of assessment that has been suggested is the 12-minute walking test (p. 43) before and after nebulised bronchodilators.[12]

An electric air compressor is the most convenient means of powering a nebuliser in the home as it is portable and gives the

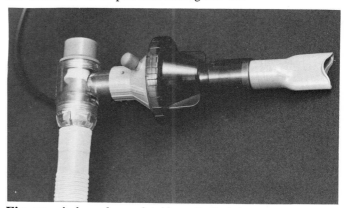

Fig. 79. *Ambu valve and tubing attached to Bird micronebuliser.*

incapacitated patient who is dependent on this form of treatment the possibility of making visits away from home. Arrangements must be made to have compressors regularly serviced.

The standard British domiciliary flow head fitted to an oxygen cylinder is unsuitable as the driving source for a nebuliser, as it has a maximum output of only 4 litres per minute. A flow meter permitting higher flows of oxygen must be supplied if this is to be the driving source for a nebuliser at home.

Cleaning and sterilisation

Nebulisers must be rinsed after each treatment, and the jets probed at frequent intervals. Sterilisation should be carried out as with IPPB equipment (p. 102).

HUMIDIFICATION

During normal respirations the inspired air is warmed and humidified by the mucous membranes, so that it is fully saturated at body temperature when it reaches the trachea. If with disease there is fever, hyperventilation or dehydration, the mucosa of the upper airways may become dehydrated. If there is not sufficient moisture available to replace that used up in humidifying the inspired air, ciliary activity is decreased, because efficient action of the cilia is dependent on continuous moistening of the respiratory mucosa (p. 4). Dehydration also makes bronchial secretions become thick and viscid. The combination of these tenacious secretions with depressed ciliary activity makes expectoration difficult.

Distressed breathless patients often do not drink enough and if fluids are given by mouth or infusion, the secretions will become less tenacious. Humidification of the inspired air or oxygen may also assist in loosening secretions and aid expectoration.

When the upper respiratory tract is by-passed by means of an endotracheal tube or tracheostomy tube, humidification of the inspired gases is essential to prevent drying and crusting of the secretions.

Humidity can be obtained in two different ways: either by inhaling water vapour, or inhaling a mist of nebulised particles.

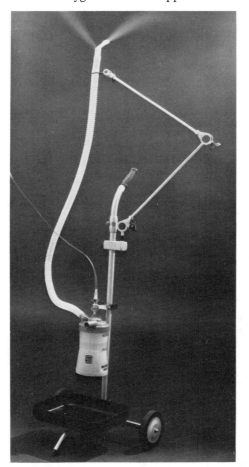

Fig. 80. *Solo-Sphere Nebuliser powered by oxygen.*

The first method is the principle of the hot water humidifiers such as the East-Radcliffe blower assisted humidifier, or the Cape humidifier. Gas is blown over the heated water and it absorbs water vapour which is then inhaled by the patient.

Nebulisers produce a mist of particles which are suspended in a stream of gas and then inhaled. Small nebulisers with a high output (p. 103) can be used for humidification, but large volume nebulisers are often more convenient. Examples of these are the Solo-sphere nebuliser (figs. 80 and 81), the Puritan all-purpose nebuliser, Bard Inspiron nebuliser, the Ohio deluxe nebuliser, and the Bird 500 ml nebuliser. Ultrasonic nebulisers also fall into this category producing a dense mist of very fine particles which may possibly be inhaled further into the respiratory tract than those producing larger particles (fig. 82).

Several humidifiers combine the features of both these methods of humidification, providing a heated vapour in which the nebulised particles are suspended. Some patients have an adverse reaction to cold air and may prefer heated humidity.

Most of these humidifiers can be incorporated into the ventilator circuit if extra humidity is required when using IPPB.

Devices which just bubble the inspired gas through cold water are not an effective means of humidification.

INDICATIONS FOR HUMIDIFICATION

1 Intubated patients

Humidification incorporated into the ventilator circuit is essential for patients undergoing artificial ventilation. When being weaned from the ventilator, adequate humidification of the inspired gases is

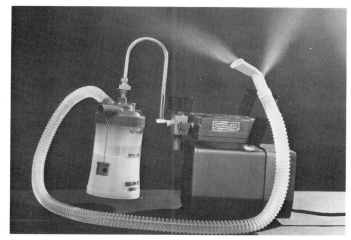

Fig. 81. *Solo-Sphere Nebuliser powered by Medic-Aid C50 compressor.*

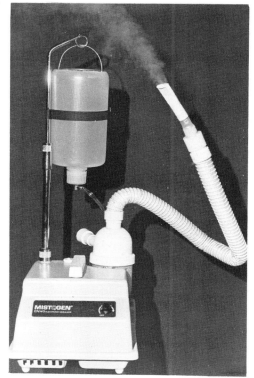

Fig. 82. *Mistogen ultrasonic nebuliser.*

equally important (p. 92). These gases are usually passed over some form of hot water humidifier and reach the tracheostomy via a special connection such as the Gilston cigar or box, or Hudson tracheostomy mask.

Occasionally a totally different type of humidifier is employed for an adult being weaned from a ventilator. It is a vapour condenser humidifier. The metal mesh or paper filter, incorporated in the device, picks up the warmth and moisture of the exhaled air as it passes through to the atmosphere and as the next breath is inhaled through the device, the air absorbs the warmth and moisture from the mesh and passes into the lungs. This method may only be satisfactory for very limited periods and will only be effective if the patient is well hydrated. The advantage is that the patient can be mobile and independent of machinery.

2 Post–operative sputum retention

If a patient is wearing a mask giving an oxygen concentration of 40% or more, one of the large volume nebulisers with high density output such as the Solo-sphere, or Ohio nebuliser with an external heater, can be connected by wide bore tubing to the mask to provide effective humidification.

Intermittent inhalations by mouth from any of the humidifiers previously mentioned, are often helpful preceding assisted coughing or postural drainage. Simple steam inhalations can be useful provided the patient inspires deeply and precautions are taken to avoid spillage.

3 Infants and children

It is particularly important to provide high humidity for infants and children who have thick secretions, as their small airways can easily become blocked and cause a collapse of areas of lung. If the child is too small to tolerate a mask, humidity can be provided by a head box, or the child can be nursed in a tent.

Patients particularly at risk are those who have just been extubated or those with laryngeal problems. Children with cystic fibrosis, pneumonia or bronchiolitis may need to be nursed in high humidity.

4 Tenacious secretions in medical chest disease

Inhalations of sterile water or normal saline by mouthpiece, for 10–15 minutes preceding postural drainage, are helpful in exacerbations of cystic fibrosis (p. 55), in allergic bronchopulmonary aspergillosis (p. 59), and in occasional cases of asthma with severe plugging of the airways. Humidifiers particularly successful with these conditions are ultrasonic nebulisers, or nebulisers incorporating a heating device.

Treatment can be repeated 2 hourly if necessary. It is a wise precaution to test the patient's FEV$_1$ or PEFR before and after inhaling from the humidifier, to ensure that no deterioration has been caused. The recordings after inhalation should not be taken immediately following a bout of coughing. A true reading should be obtained after the airways have had a short period to relax.

5 Humidification with controlled oxygen therapy

Many patients who require controlled oxygen therapy, such as a chronic bronchitic with an acute exacerbation, have viscid tenacious secretions. Controlled oxygen is often provided by means of a Ventimask connected to the oxygen supply by a narrow bore tube. Effective humidification via narrow bore tubing is impossible due to condensation.

A device known as a humidity adapter can be used, whereby the air entrained by the mask is humidified. It is a cuff which partially surrounds the air entraining holes of the Ventimask (fig. 83), and is connected by a wide bore tubing to a humidifier. The humidifier must be powered by an air source. This can be piped air if it is available, an air cylinder or an electric air compressor capable of continuous use (e.g. Medic-Aid Hush-Pump).

A nebuliser such as the Solo-sphere, Puritan or Inspiron (fig. 84) can be used. High humidification is obtained if this type of nebuliser is powered by 6–8 litres of air per minute and the air entrainment control of the nebuliser itself is adjusted to give maximum flow of humidified air to the patient. A hot-water humidifier such as the Cape can be used with a high flow of air across it. The flow of air from the humidifier to the patient must be at least 10 litres per minute and then humidification of the inspired gases is greatly improved without altering the percentage of oxygen delivered.[13]

6 Sputum specimens

It is frequently important that specimens of sputum should be obtained for diagnostic purposes, for example in suspected bronchial carcinoma. If no secretions are produced despite breathing exercises, huffing and coughing, it may be helpful to inhale hypertonic saline from an ultrasonic nebuliser. 7% saline (1·21 M) has been found to enhance clearance of bronchial secretions.[14]

A few millilitres of hypertonic saline are placed in the 'medicine cup' of the ultrasonic nebuliser. The patient inhales for 5–10 minutes and is often able to expectorate bronchial secretions.

If an ultrasonic nebuliser is not available, a small nebuliser producing an aerosol of fine particle size may be as effective.

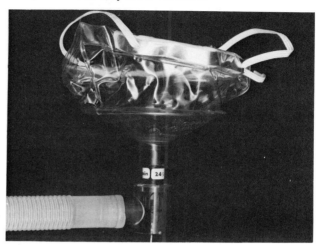

Fig. 83. *Ventimask with humidity adapter.*

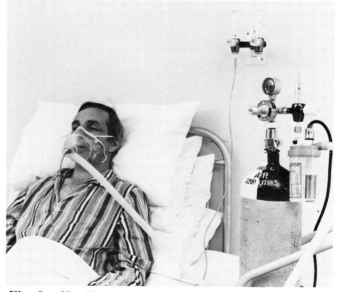

Fig. 84. *Humidity adapter in use with Bard Inspiron Nebuliser.*

Sterilisation of equipment

It is important to sterilise all humidifiers regularly to prevent re-infection. Unlike IPPB machines where it is only necessary to sterilise the breathing-head assembly, humidifiers must be sterilised entirely before being used by another patient.

References

1. OPIE L.H. & SPALDING J.M.K. (1958) Chest physiotherapy during intermittent positive-pressure respiration. *Lancet* ii, 671.
2. CLEMENT A.J. & HÜBSCH S.K. (1968) Chest physiotherapy by the 'bag squeezing' method. *Physiotherapy* **54,** (10), 355.
3. GORMEZANO J. & BRANTHWAITE M.A. (1972) Effects of physiotherapy during intermittent positive pressure ventilation. *Anaesthesia* **27,** 258.
4. BRANTHWAITE M.A. (1978) *Artificial Ventilation for Pulmonary Disease.* Pitman Medical, Tonbridge, Kent.
5. SYKES M.K., McNICOL M.W. & CAMPBELL E.J.M. (1976) *Respiratory Failure.* 2nd edition. Blackwell Scientific Publications, Oxford.
6. AYRES S.M., KOZAM R.L. & LUKAS D.S. (1963) The effects of intermittent positive pressure breathing on intrathoracic pressure, pulmonary mechanics and the work of breathing. *American Review of Respiratory Disease* **87,** 370.
7. SUKUMALCHANTRA Y., PARK S.S. & WILLIAMS M.H. (1965) Effect of intermittent positive pressure breathing (IPPB) in acute ventilatory failure. *American Review of Respiratory Disease* **92,** 885.
8. GORMEZANO J. & BRANTHWAITE M.A. (1972) Pulmonary physiotherapy with assisted ventilation. *Anaesthesia* **27,** 249.
9. SHENFIELD G.M., EVANS M.E. & PATERSON J.W. (1974) The effect of different nebulisers with and without intermittent positive pressure breathing on the absorption and metabolism of salbutamol. *British Journal of Clinical Pharmacology* **1,** 295.
10. WOLFSDORF J., SWIFT D.L. & AVERY M.E. (1969) Mist therapy reconsidered; an evaluation of the respiratory deposition of labelled water aerosols produced by jet and ultrasonic nebulisers. *Pediatrics* **43,** 799.
11. HOWARD P., CAYTON R.M., BRENNAN S.R. & ANDERSON P.B. (1977) Lignocaine aerosol and persistent cough. *British Journal of Diseases of the Chest* **71,** 19.
12. WILSON R.S.E. (1979) Salbutamol by compressor driven nebuliser in domiciliary use. *Journal of Pharmacotherapy* **2,** 65.
13. WEBBER B.A. (1976) Humidification with controlled oxygen therapy. *Physiotherapy* **62,** (6), 192.
14. PAVIA D., THOMSON M.L. & CLARKE S.W. (1978) Enhanced clearance of secretions from the human lung after the administration of hypertonic saline aerosol. *American Review of Respiratory Disease* **117,** 199.

9 Paediatric cardiothoracic surgery

PULMONARY SURGERY

Pulmonary surgery is rarely performed in infants, but when it is necessary the principles of physiotherapy are the same as for cardiac surgery. For older children undergoing pulmonary surgery, treatment is similar to that for adults.

CARDIAC SURGERY FOR INFANTS AND CHILDREN

Paediatric cardiac surgery is a rapidly expanding speciality and many advances in technique have been made. The majority of infants and children undergoing cardiac surgery have congenital cardiac defects. Some of the more commonly performed operations include: ligation of patent ductus arteriosus, resection of coarctation of the aorta, open pulmonary or aortic valvotomy, closure of atrial and ventricular septal defects, total correction of Fallot's tetralogy, Mustard's operation for transposition of the great arteries and correction of anomalous pulmonary venous drainage.

Certain palliative operations such as banding of the pulmonary artery or various shunts may also be performed.

PRE-OPERATIVE TRAINING

The amount of pre-operative training possible in children naturally depends on their age. As well as teaching the child, it is important to explain the necessity of the exercises to the parents who are often with the children for long periods of the day and can encourage practice.

Infants

Infants with cardiac defects often suffer from pulmonary hypertension and frequently have excessive secretions and are prone to repeated chest infections. It may be necessary to give physiotherapy pre-operatively to clear the chest. This consists of modified postural drainage, percussion or gentle vibrations and naso-pharyngeal suction to stimulate coughing.

18 months–3 years

It is usually possible to teach deep breathing by means of blowing bubbles or paper tissues. If bronchial secretions are present pre-operatively, postural drainage can probably be performed (with the doctor's permission) and percussion over the chest usually induces coughing.

3 years upwards

Diaphragmatic breathing, lower thoracic expansion exercises and coughing can be taught. Possibly up to the age of 5, the incentive of blowing bubbles or paper tissues may be necessary. Postural drainage can be performed if required.

Arm movements may be encouraged by clapping the hands over the head and for children over 5 years old, more shoulder girdle and arm exercises are included.

POST-OPERATIVE TREATMENT

Intermittent Positive Pressure Ventilation

If the infant is artificially ventilated, physiotherapy may be requested. Gentle percussion or chest vibrations and suction are given in a side-lying position, if possible. Manual hyperinflation may possibly be indicated (p. 88), but this should only be carried out by experienced staff because of the dangers of causing a pneumothorax.

Saline (0·5 ml for a small baby) can be instilled before manual inflation. If it is inserted into the top of the endotracheal (or tracheostomy) tube, very little may reach the bronchi because of the small volume. It is often more effective to fill a catheter with saline and, leaving the syringe attached, insert it into the endotracheal tube as far as it will go, withdraw it 1 cm (to ensure that it is above the carina), and then instil a further 0·5 ml of saline.

An infant's airways are so narrow that a

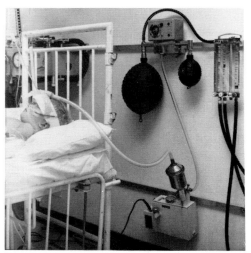

Fig. 85. *Continuous positive airways pressure system in use. By courtesy of* Anaesthesia.

small amount of mucus can block off a large area of lung tissue and rapid deterioration in the patient's condition may occur. Efficient, quick and regular suction is essential for any infant nursed on a ventilator.

The treatment of older children undergoing I P P V is similar to that of adults (p. 88).

Continuous Positive Airways Pressure

Continuous positive airways pressure (CPAP) is used in the management of infants suffering from respiratory distress syndrome and is being increasingly used for infants and children following cardiac surgery. In the latter case, it provides a useful transition between I P P V and extubation and may permit earlier weaning from a ventilator. The patient breathes spontaneously against continuous positive pressure.

It is probable that CPAP assists in keeping the airways patent. It has been shown that following cardiac surgery in infants, the functional residual capacity (FRC) is reduced and that CPAP causes the FRC to rise towards the normal.[1] When compliance is reduced following open heart surgery, it has been shown that CPAP results in a significant increase in Pao_2.

There are various CPAP systems in use. The one currently used at Brompton Hospital is compact and incorporates a safety system and hand ventilation device.[2] It utilises a constant gas flow and an adjustable leak to produce the desired pressure. The system (fig. 85) includes a reservoir bag, pressure gauge, high and low pressure warning device, adjustable blow-off valve, 500 ml bag for hand ventilation, heated humidifier and a single line to the patient with the adjustable leak 'at the mouth' (fig. 86).

Pressures are set initially at about 10 cm

H_2O and over a period of time are decreased to 1–2 cm H_2O at which point the child is extubated.

Physiotherapy for these patients is similar to that used for those undergoing IPPV. If manual hyperinflation is to be used, it can either be done via a separate circuit, or using the 500 ml bag in the CPAP circuit.

If the latter system is used, the outlet of the adjustable leak on the end piece is partially occluded with a fingertip during inspiration to give sufficient inflation pressure.

The technique of manual hyperinflation should only be carried out by experienced staff. Hyperinflation should be synchronised with the patient's inspiratory effort and pressure should not be excessive because of the risk of pneumothorax.

When positioning these patients, it is important to ensure that the tubing is maintained in a dependent position behind the child's head, otherwise condensation from the humidified gases could drain into the respiratory tract.

Since an infant's breathing is predominantly diaphragmatic, the child should be positioned to ensure free movement of the diaphragm.

Not all patients undergoing CPAP require regular physiotherapy. Some patients may only have minimal secretions which can easily be cleared by regular suction and change of position. In these cases, there is no point in carrying out physiotherapy and subjecting the child to unnecessary discomfort. It is, however, very important for the physiotherapist, at frequent intervals, to ascertain that the patient's condition remains satisfactory, as the situation can change very rapidly.

After the child has been extubated, physiotherapy is continued at regular intervals, possibly two hourly. The child is placed in side-lying and if necessary tipped and the chest percussed; coughing is encouraged in this position, naso-pharyngeal suction may be necessary for those unable to cough to command. If the patient's respirations are inadequate and there is not a satisfactory response to this type of treatment, assisted ventilation should be given by means of a mask and bag.[3] The mask is held tightly over the face and the neck is extended with the chin up. Assisted ventilation is normally given with the patient in the supine position, but during physiotherapy, it may be necessary to turn the child into side-lying. It is very important to synchronise with the patient's inspiratory phase, otherwise the stomach will become inflated. This technique should only be carried out by experienced staff.

Where collapse of part or the whole of a lung has occurred and is not responding to physiotherapy, this may be treated by temporary intubation in order to permit efficient inflation and suction during physiotherapy.

Older children may respond well to IPPB with a mask or mouthpiece and this can be

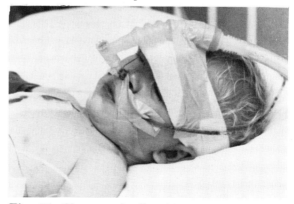

Fig. 86. *Close up of adjustable end-piece in CPAP system. By courtesy of* Anaesthesia.

carried out successfully in conjunction with physiotherapy.

Post–operative treatment of non–intubated patients

Older children will be treated in a similar manner to adults (p 83).

Younger children should be turned into side-lying and gentle pressure given to the chest wall to encourage expansion. Percussion may be helpful in stimulating a cough; the child can be 'tipped' if the doctor gives permission.

Spontaneous coughing is often induced with crying; but if the breath sounds are diminished, secretions are present, and the child will not cough spontaneously, some other means of stimulating a cough must be used.

In children, the trachea is soft and mobile, so that intermittent lateral pressure on the trachea with a finger tip, produces apposition of the tracheal walls resulting in instant stimulation of the cough reflex.

Small babies will require naso-pharyngeal suction, and this may also be necessary in older children if other methods fail.

Many infants and children are nursed in high humidity for the immediate post-operative period as it is important that secretions do not become thick and occlude the small airways.

If the cardiac condition is stable, small children are often allowed out of bed and the additional mobility will stimulate deep breathing and coughing.

Many children have no problems with chest secretions after cardiac surgery. Some may develop very poor posture and are reluctant to move, in which case, suitable exercises should be given.

References

1. GREGORY G A., EDMUNDS L H., KITTERMAN J.A., PHIBBS R.H. & TOOLEY W.H. (1975) Continuous positive airway pressure and pulmonary and circulatory function after cardiac surgery in infants less than three months of age. *Anesthesiology* **43,** 426.

2. PFITZNER J., BRANTHWAITE M.A., ENGLISH I.C.W. & SHINEBOURNE E.A. (1974) Continuous positive airway pressure. *Anaesthesia* **29,** 326.

3. GREGORY G.A. (1972) Respiratory care of newborn infants. *Pediatric Clinics of North America* **19,** 311.

Suggested reading list

1. *Principles of Chest X-Ray Diagnosis* (1978) 4th edition. G.SIMON. Butterworths, London.
2. *Lung Sounds* (1978) P. FORGACS. Ballière Tindall, London.
3. *Respiratory Physiology—the essentials* (1974) J.B. WEST. Williams and Wilkins, Baltimore.
4. *Pulmonary Pathophysiology—the essentials* (1977) J.B. WEST. Williams and Wilkins, Baltimore.
5. *The Respiratory Muscles* (1970) 2nd edition. E.J.M. CAMPBELL, E.AGOSTONI & J.NEWSOM DAVIS. Lloyd-Luke, London.
6. *Respiratory Function in Disease.* (1971) 2nd edition. D.V. BATES, P.T.MACKLEM & R.V.CHRISTIE. Saunders, Philadelphia.
7. *Respiratory Failure* (1976) 2nd edition. M.K.SYKES, M.W.McNICOL & E.J.M. CAMPBELL. Blackwell Scientific Publications, Oxford.
8. *Respiratory Diseases* (1975) 2nd edition. J.CROFTON & A.DOUGLAS. Blackwell Scientific Publications, Oxford.
9. *Disorders of the Respiratory System* (1979) 2nd edition. G.CUMMING & S.J.SEMPLE. Blackwell Scientific Publications, Oxford.
10. *A Synopsis of Chest Diseases* (1979) J.V.COLLINS. Wright, Bristol.
11. *Asthma* (1977) Eds. T.J.H.CLARK & S.GODFREY. Chapman and Hall, London.
12. *The Natural History of Chronic Bronchitis and Emphysema* (1976) C.FLETCHER, R.PETO, C.TINKER & F.E.SPEIZER. Oxford University Press, Oxford.
13. *The Pathology of Emphysema* (1967) L.REID. Lloyd-Luke, London.
14. *Cystic Fibrosis, Manual of Diagnosis and Management* (1976) C.M.ANDERSON & M.C.GOODCHILD. Blackwell Scientific Publications, Oxford.
15. *Pulmonary Disease of the Fetus, Newborn and Child* (1978) E.M.SCARPELLI, P.A.M.AULD, H.S.GOLDMAN. Lea and Febiger, Philadelphia.
16. *Current Paediatric Cardiology* (1980) E.A. SHINEBOURNE & R.H. ANDERSON. Oxford University Press, Oxford.
17. *A Synopsis of Cardiology* (1979) 2nd edition. S.C.JORDAN. Wright, Bristol.
18. *Intensive Care of the Heart and Lungs: a Text for Nurses* (1975) 2nd edition. E.A.HARRIS, J.M.NEUTZE, M.P.RICKARD, E.R.SEELYE & M.M.SIMPSON. Blackwell Scientific Publications, Oxford.
19. *Artificial Ventilation for Pulmonary Disease* (1980) 2nd edition. M.A. BRANTHWAITE. Pitman Medical, Tonbridge, Kent.
20. *Clinical Pharmacology* (1980) 5th edition. D.R.LAURENCE & P.N.BENNETT. Churchill Livingstone, Edinburgh.

Index